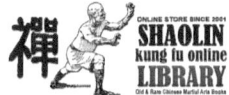
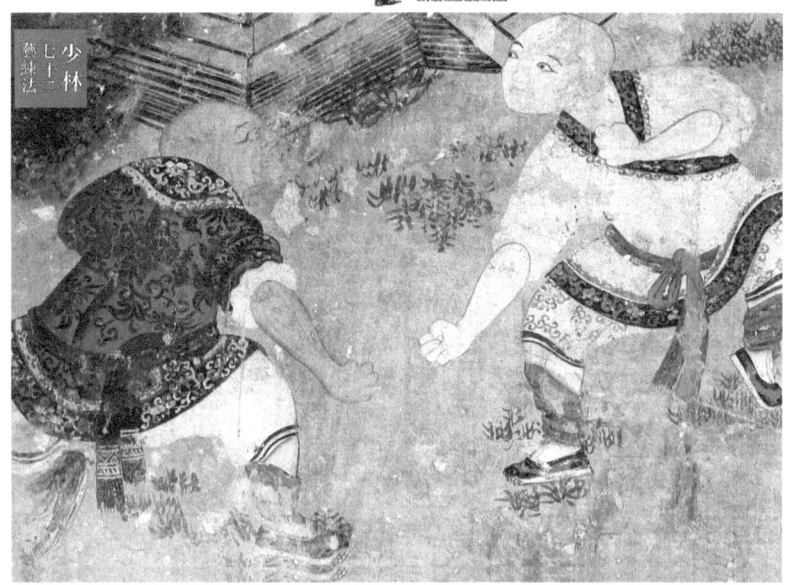
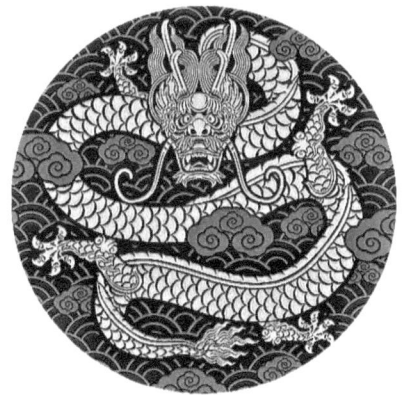

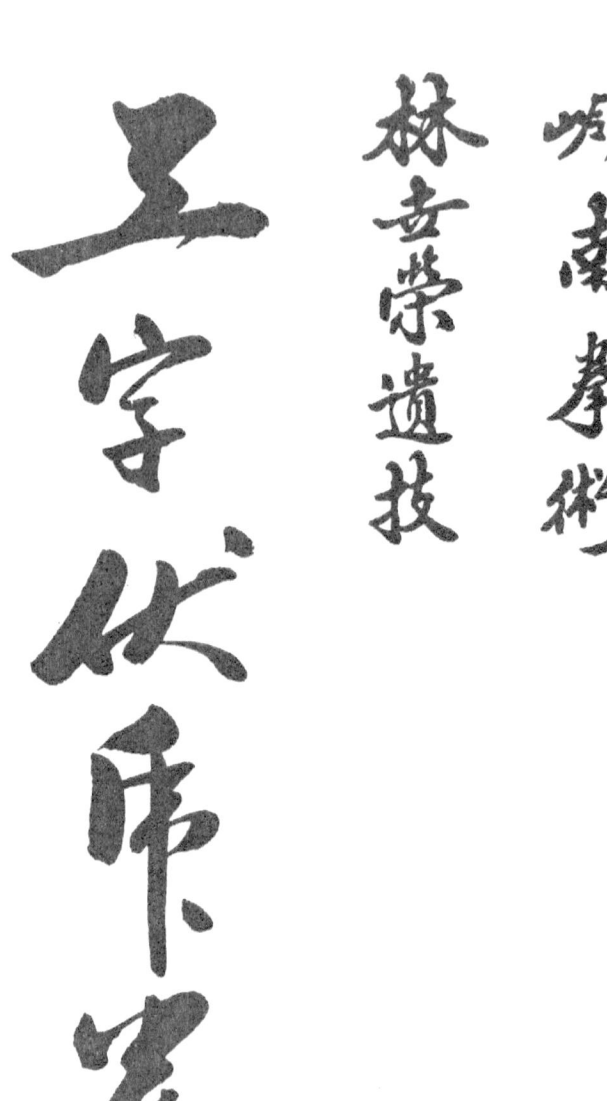

嶺南拳術

林世榮遺技

工字伏虎拳

林世榮著

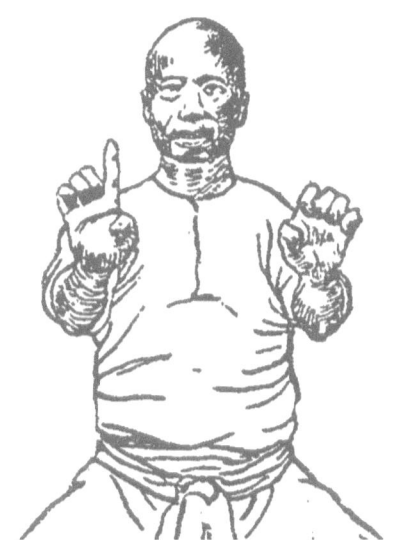

SOUTHERN SHAOLIN HUNG GAR KUNG FU
CLASSICS SERIES

TAMING the TIGER

Priceless Heritage of Southern Shaolin
Inherited from the Past and Handed Down by Venerable Grandmaster
Lam Sai Wing

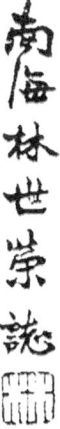

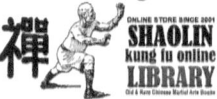
LAM SAI WING.
TAMING THE TIGER. SOUTHERN SHAOLIN HUNG GAR
KUNG FU CLASSICS SERIES

*The book scrutinizes an old canonical form (Tao Lu) of Southern
Shaolin Kung Fu, the "Taming the Tiger Fist" (工字伏虎拳, 'Gung
Gee Fook Fu Kuen'). According to surviving sources, the founder of
the Hung Gar style, Luk Ah Choy (陸阿采), studied this form under
the tutorship of Southern Shaolin's best fighter, a Grandmaster of the
White Tiger Style Southern Shaolin abbot Gee Sin Sim Si (至善禪師).*

Shaolin Kung Fu Online Library

**Chinese Martial Arts - Theory & Practice / Old & Rare Chinese
Books, Treatises, Manuscripts**

www.shaolinkungfulibrary.com

/Old and Rare Chinese Books in English/

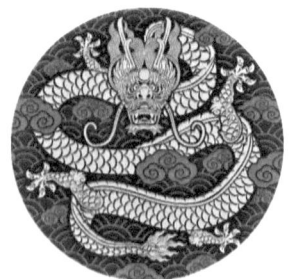

Shaolin Kung Fu Online Library

2025

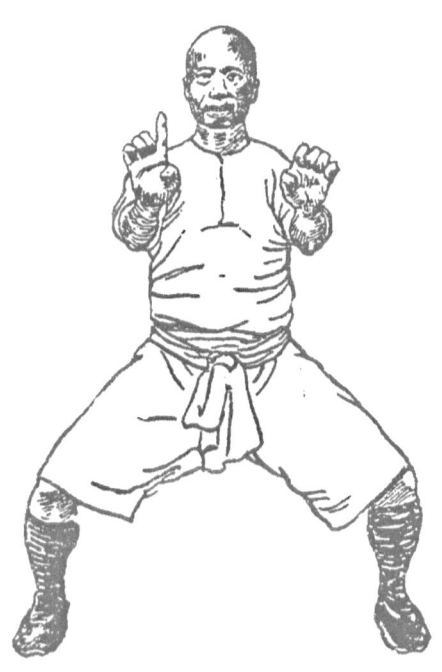

TAMING *the* TIGER

SOUTHERN SHAOLIN
HUNG GAR KUNG FU CLASSICS SERIES

SECOND, REVISED AND UPDATED EDITION

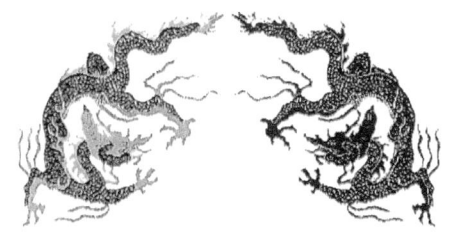

Lam Sai Wing

Andrew Timofeevich (Translator)

Shaolin Kung Fu Online Library

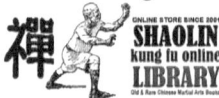

shaolinkungfulibrary.com

Southern Shaolin Hung Gar Kung Fu Classics Series:

Lam Sai Wing, Taming the Tiger.
Lam Sai Wing, Tiger and Crane.
Lam Sai Wing, Iron Thread.

TAMING THE TIGER. SOUTHERN SHAOLIN HUNG GAR KUNG FU CLASSICS SERIES

Second, Revised and Updated Edition

First Edition: Lam Sai Wing, Andrew Timofeevich. *Gung Gee Fook Fu Kuen. Moving Along the Hieroglyph GUNG, I Tame the Tiger with the Pugilistic Art* (*eBook*, Shaolin Kung Fu Online Library, 2002).

Compiled and edited by Andrew Timofeevich. Translated by Andrew Timofeevich, Wang Ke Ze, Leonid Serbin, and Oleg Korshunov. Commentaries: Andrew Timofeevich.

Book design by Andrew Timofeevich and Olga Akimova.

Published by Shaolin Kung Fu Online Library

USA, 2025

ISBN: 979-8-218-88890-9

www.shaolinkungfulibrary.com

Disclaimer:

The author and publisher of this material are not responsible in any manner whatsoever for any injury that may occur through reading or following the instructions in this manual. The physical or otherwise activities described in this material may be too strenuous or dangerous for some people, and the reader should consult a physician before engaging in them.

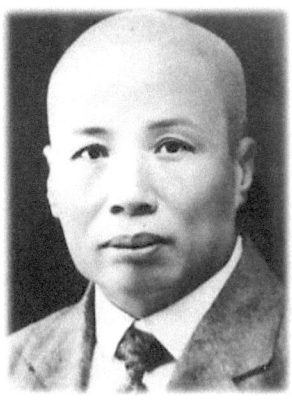

Venerable Grandmaster

Lam Sai Wing

(1860 – 1943)

"Since my young years till now, for 50 years, I have been learning from Masters. I am happy that I have earned the love of my tutors who passed on me the Shaolin Mastery..."

"This book will help to reach the mastership in Fighting Art that is not simple to understand. It has been written with the aim of handing down the knowledge to disciples who are eager to find tutors and expect to receive instructions."

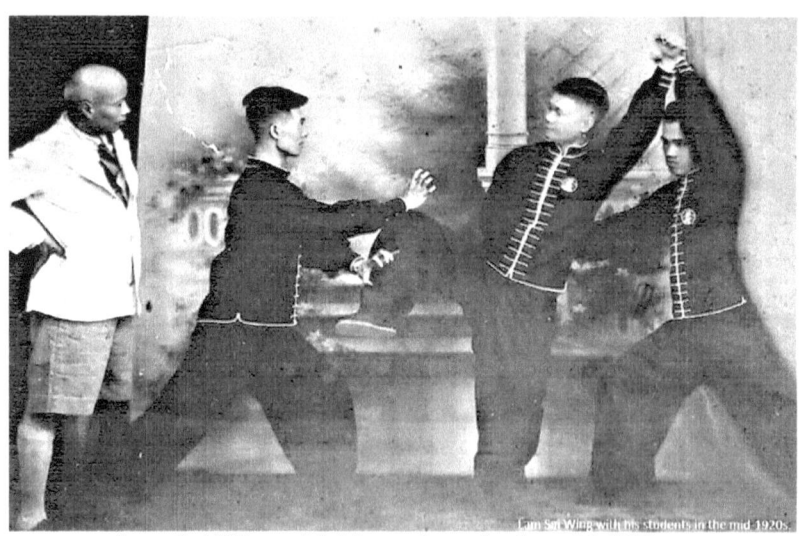
Lam Sai Wing with his students in the mid-1920s.

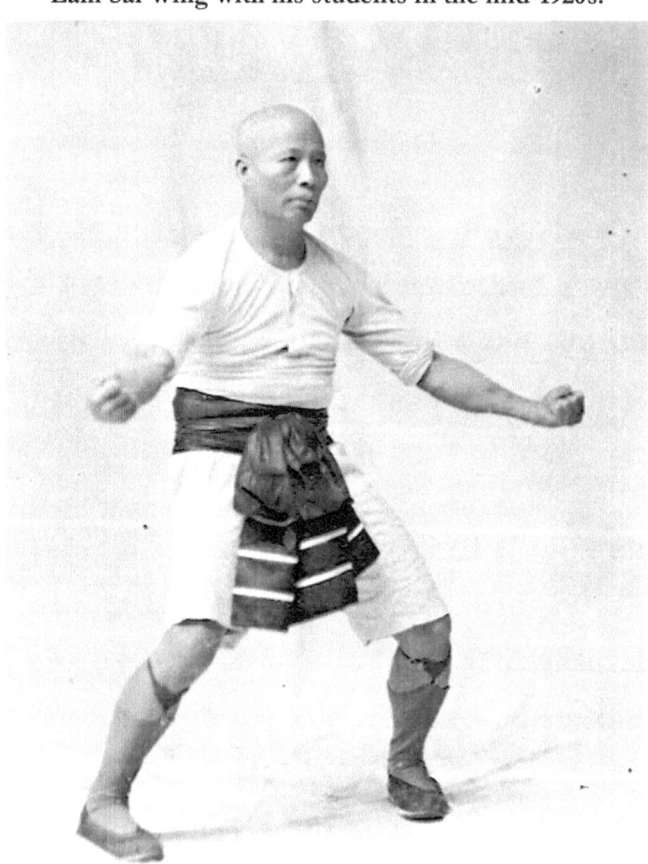
Lam Sai Wing performs a technique called "Dividing the Gold Bridge" (分金橋, Cantonese: *FAN GAM KIU*).

About the Author[I]

Lam Sai Wing (1861 - 1943) was born in the district of *Nan Hai*, *Guangdong* province. Followed the customs of ancestors and learnt the tradition of Martial Arts in his family, proceeded to learn from tutors *Lam Fook Sing*, *Wong Fei Hung*, and *Wu Gum Sin*.

Indulged in persistent training, achieved great mastership in the Martial Arts. Founded *Wu Ben Tang* ("The Hall of Fundamental Study") in *Guangzhou (Canton)* where he taught the Martial Arts. During his life brought up more than 10,000 followers.

Toward the end of the *Qing* dynasty (1644 - 1911), *Lam Sai Wing* gained the first place at large competitions that took place at the *Dongjiao* ground. Thanks to this, with great pleasure, *Lam Sai Wing* received a silver medal handed to him by *Dr. Sun Yat-Sen*[II] himself as a token of the recognition of his great services and successes.

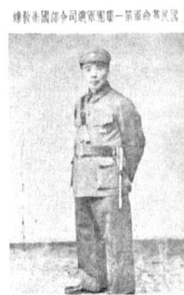

Lam Sai Wing while serving as a hand-to-hand combat training inspector at the Headquarters of The New 1st Army (新一軍, nicknamed the *"First Army under Heaven"*) of the Chinese National Revolutionary Army (probably the second half of the 1920s).

[I] An article from *ZHONG GUO WU SHU ZEN MING CI DIAN* - Dictionary "Well-known Masters of the Chinese Wu Shu" edited by Chang Cang and Zhou Li Chang.

[II] *Sun Yat-Sen* (his other names: *Sun Zhongshan*, Sun Wen) (1866 - 1925), a Chinese revolutionary democrat, the leader of the Chinese Revolution of 1911 - 1913, the first (provisional) president of the Chinese Republic (1 January - 1 April, 1912). In 1912 founded *Guomindang* party.

In the years followed, taking images and characters of the Tiger and the Crane as a base, as well as techniques of *Hung Gar Kuen*[III] and *Fo Kuen*[IV] styles, he founded a new school *Fu Hok Seung Ying Kuen* ("The Double Form of the Tiger and the Crane").

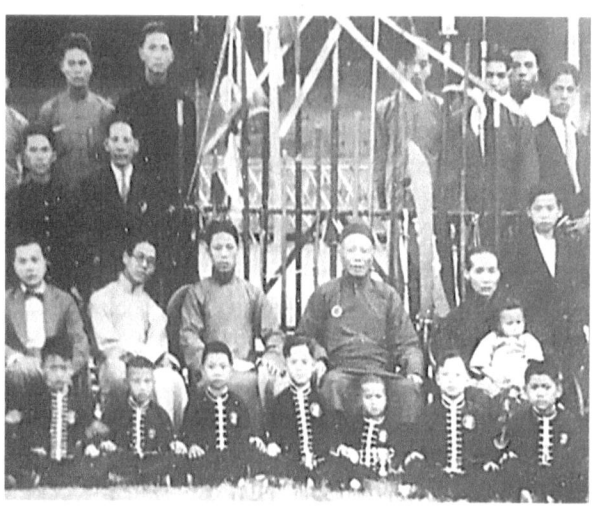

Lam Sai Wing with his nephew Lam Cho (to the left of him) and students (Hong Kong, 1932)

Lived in his old years in *Hong Kong* where he taught the Martial Arts together with his favorite disciples *Juy Yu Jaai*, *Jeung Sai Biu*, *Lei Sai Fai*, and others. Wrote books: *GUNG GEE FOOK FU KUEN* ("Taming the Tiger"), *TID SIN KUEN* ("Iron Thread Fist"), and *FU HOK SEUNG YING KUEN* ("The Double Form of the Tiger and the Crane").

Marked a new epoch and a new school of Chinese Martial Arts, particularly in the division of formal complexes *Tao Lu*. *Fu Hok Seung Ying Kuen* is practiced on a large scale both in China and abroad, and interest in it does not fall down. After the

---

[III] *Hung Gar Kuen* - "The Fist of Hung Family". This style was widespread in secret societies *Gelaohui* ("The union of the Elder Brother"), *Sandianhui* ("The Triad"), and others in the Southern China in the XIX - the beginning of the XX century. It is remarkable for its very high fighting efficiency. It takes its origin from the Southern Shaolin Tiger style.

[IV] *Fo Kuen* - "The fist of Buddhist brotherhood" was practised in secret Buddhist sects in *Guangdong* province. That style also originates from the Southern Shaolin.

formation of the People's Republic of China (1949) this style was included into syllabuses of institutes and *Wu Shu* high-grade schools.

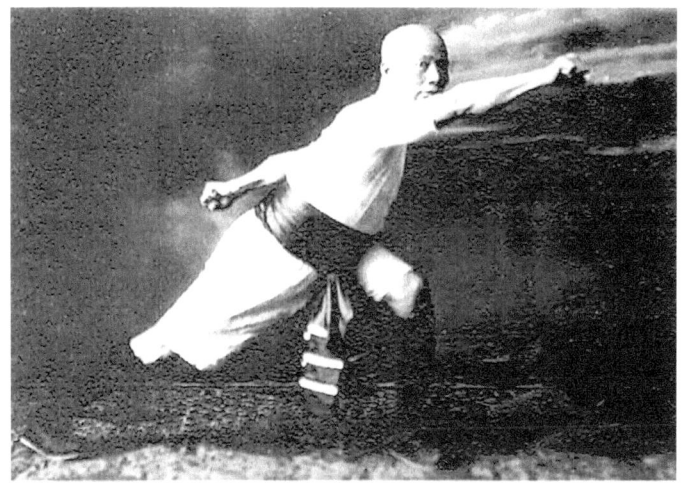

Lam Sai Wing performs a technique called "Beat the Drum with a Stone Pestle" (碌鼓搥, Cantonese: *LUK GU CEOI*).

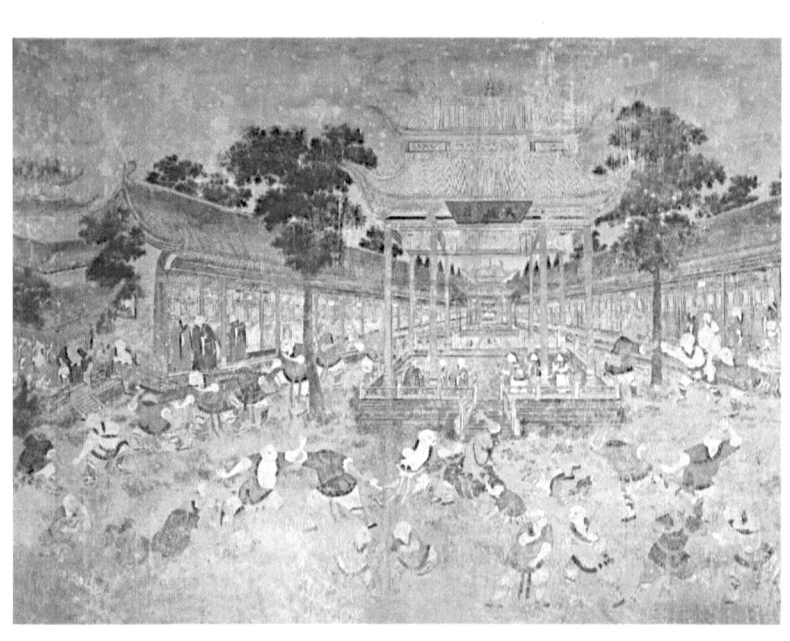

Contents

Preface by the Author

During the reign of the *Qing* Emperor *Yongzheng* (雍正, 1722-1735), the Japanese invaded *Taiwan*. When the news about the Japanese seizure of some towns reached the *Qing* Government, it was terrified and sent the Chinese troops to take back the island. However, the Chinese army suffered defeat after defeat, and military commanders of different ranks were not able to drive the Japanese away.

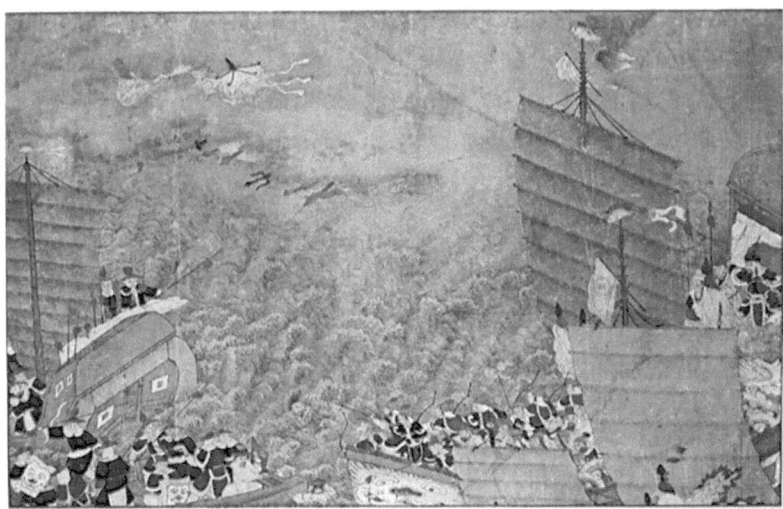

A naval battle between Japanese pirates and the Chinese. (18th Century, China).

After that, a detachment of monks from the *Shaolin* Monastery in *Fujian* province came to *Taiwan*. Full of audacity and courage, they delivered a decisive blow to the Japanese invaders. The Japanese suffered a defeat and retreated. *Taiwan* was liberated.

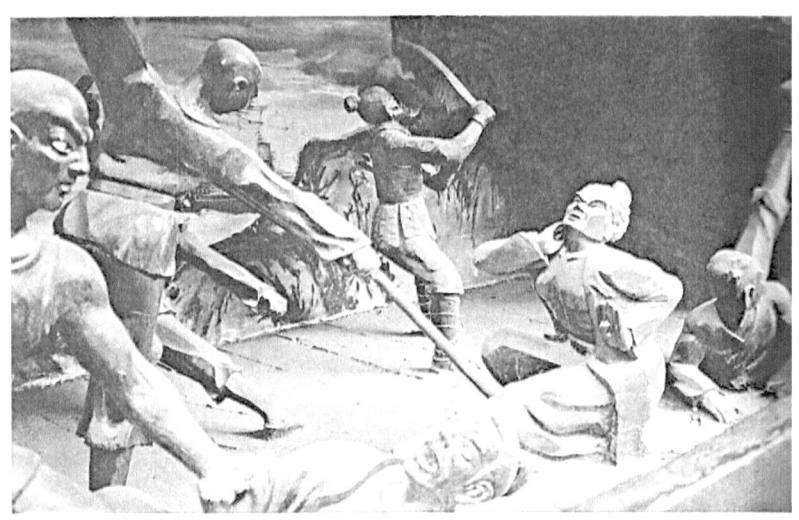

Shaolin monks engaged in a fight with Japanese invaders. Gallery of wooden sculptures at the Shaolin Monastery.

The *Qing* Government rejoiced over the victory and intended to grant various titles and posts to the most courageous monks. However, the unworldly Buddhist monks did not accept granted posts, so they were awarded land allotments to grow rice and other valuable presents.

The *Qing* bureaucracy thought that if there were such outstanding persons in the *Shaolin* Monastery, they might be dangerous to the Emperor's Palace. If anti-*Qing* feelings become strong among the monks, it could be very harmful. The *Qing* Government sent to the monks grain and presents. At the same time some people sent by the government secretly brought to the walls of the monastery a lot of straw. One night, a fire broke out that completely ruined the Southern *Shaolin* Monastery.

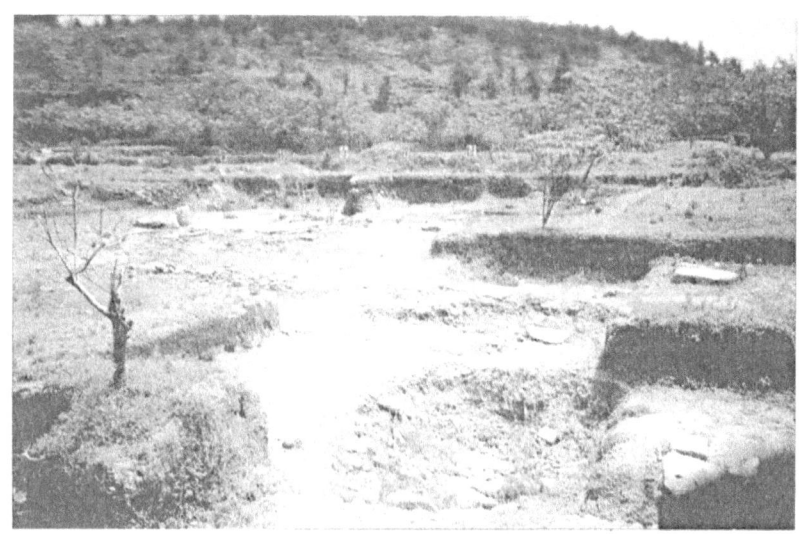

The Ruins of Southern Shaolin (late 20th century).

Image from the book: A.A. Maslow, *Encyclopedia of Eastern Martial Arts, Vol. 1: Traditions and Mysteries of Chinese Kung Fu.*

The monks who survived the fire scattered in different directions all over China, like "stars in the sky." One of the most esteemed monks, *Zhi Shan* (至善禪師, Cantonese: *Jee Sin Sim See*), settled in *Haichuang* Temple (海幢寺) in *Nanhai* District (南海) near the city of *Guangzhou* (廣州), *Guangdong* province. There, he started to teach monks different martial arts methods.

The most outstanding among his disciples was *Luk Ah Choy* (陸亞彩), a monk who greatly succeeded in learning. *Luk Ah Choy* handed down his skills to *Wong Tai* (黃泰, *Wong* from the village of *Louzhou* in *Nanhai* district, near the town of *Xiqiao*). *Wong Tai* handed down his skills to his son *Wong Kay Ying* (黃

麒英), *Wong Kay Ying* to his son *Wong Fei Hung* (黃飛鴻), who became a successor of the Martial Art in the fourth generation[I].

Later, *Wong Fei Hung* taught martial arts to the sailors of the *Guangdong* Navy (*Guangdong* Fleet, 廣東水師) under Admiral *Wu Quanmei* (吳全美) and served as chief hand-to-hand combat instructor in the so-called "Black Flag Army" under General *Liu Yongfu* (劉永福).

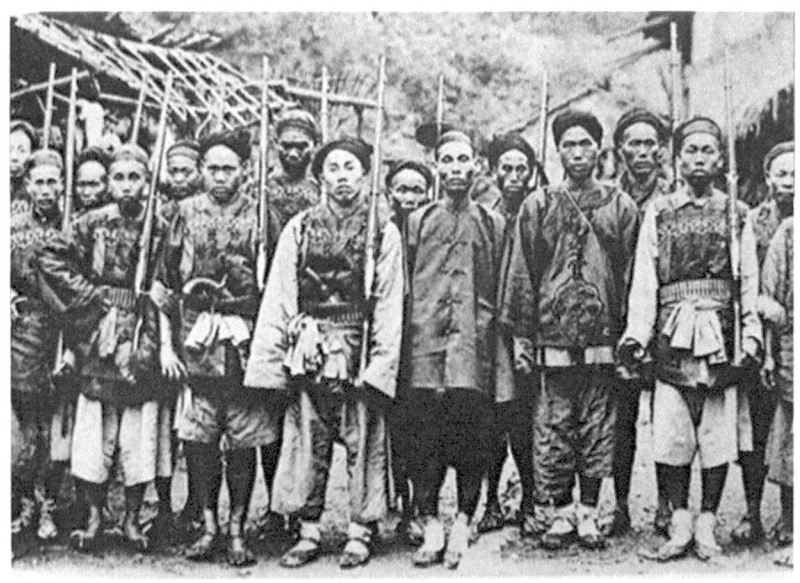

The Brave Black Flag Army Soldiers

英勇黑旗軍

[I] ***Editor's note:*** In China, it is customary to exalt the teacher and downplay one's own achievements, so although *Lam Sai Wing* was *Wong Fei Hung's* closest (and most renowned) student, he did not mention himself in the line of successors.

During the reign of the *Qing* emperor *Guangxu* (光緒, 1875-1908), *Wong Fei Hung* won a contest and was nominated for the post of *Jing Xun Da Qi Shou* (Great Bannerman for flood control). He served under the governor of *Fujian* province, *Tang Jinsong* (唐竟崧).

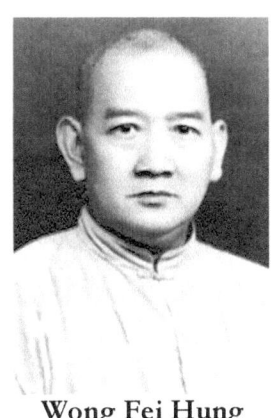

**Wong Fei Hung
(1847-1924)**

At that time, riots among common people started in *Fujian*. The people of *Fujian* province demanded that *Tang Jinsong* become the head of a democratic state and *Wong Fei Hung* be the Commander-in-chief. This news forced General *Li Hongzhang* (李鴻章) to lead a detachment of a government army of several thousand people and move out to suppress the rebellion. *Tang Jinsong* could not resist such a large force and decided to hide after shaving his mustache and beard. *Wong Fei Hung* followed *Tang Jinsong*. Both of them, without delay, fled to *Guangzhou*.

In *Guangzhou*, on *Zienan* Street, *Wong Fei Hung* established a clinic and a pharmacy named *Bo Chi Lam* (保芝林). He lived in solitude there. He did not seek any posts and did not hand down his superb skills to outsiders. A large sign was placed above the entrance with the words: *"Martial Arts are difficult to teach, and I will not pass on my knowledge even for a fortune. So do not look for a teacher here."* Therefore, those who came here in search of knowledge had no hope.

. . .

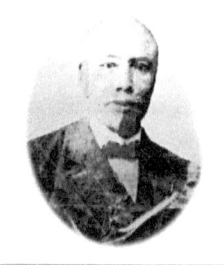

師祖林世榮先生像

工字伏虎拳略歷

清雍年間台灣被日軍佔據清政府聞報大驚傾國大小
文武將官不能取回台灣屢敗回朝偶遇福建省少林寺一班
和尚奮勇上前將日軍打退奪回台灣清政府聞報大喜欲加
封官賞因出家之人故不受封賜乐田穀米以作酬勞清政
府忽想寺內有如此能人恐防有革命之心爲害不小因起妒
忌遂於送穀米時密遣人將禾草堆積於寺側以作火引夜間
放火燒毀少林寺當時寺內各僧聞訊皆出寺逃生走得五零
星散播散各省惟至善禪師逃落粤東廣州河南海幢寺棲身
遂於寺內教授國技有陸亞彩者至善之首徒也得傳其秘而
傳與黃泰(南海西樵陸洲鄉人)黃泰傳其子麒英再傳其子
黃飛鴻是三代之祖傳黃飛鴻曾在吳全美及劉永福軍門敦
練清光緒年間在將軍衙門考得靖汛大旗手後在福建省衆
台唐竟崧部下當時福建省百姓要求唐竟崧爲民主國王黃
飛鴻遂爲殿前大將軍李鴻章統率懷軍數千餘人誅滅革命
黨起見唐竟崧不敵衆卒割鬚逃走黃飛鴻隨唐逃往廣州
市謀事不成遂在仁安街保芝林設立黃飛鴻醫館一所隱居
不傳門前大書武藝功夫難以傳授千金不傳求師莫問等語
故有志者無從問津焉

嶺南拳術

林世榮遺技

工字伏虎拳

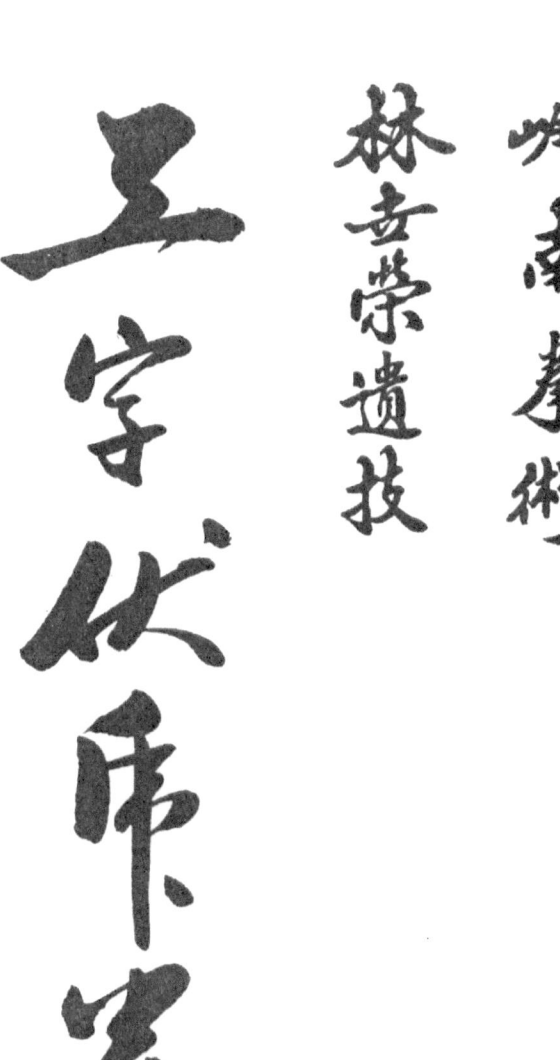

林世榮著

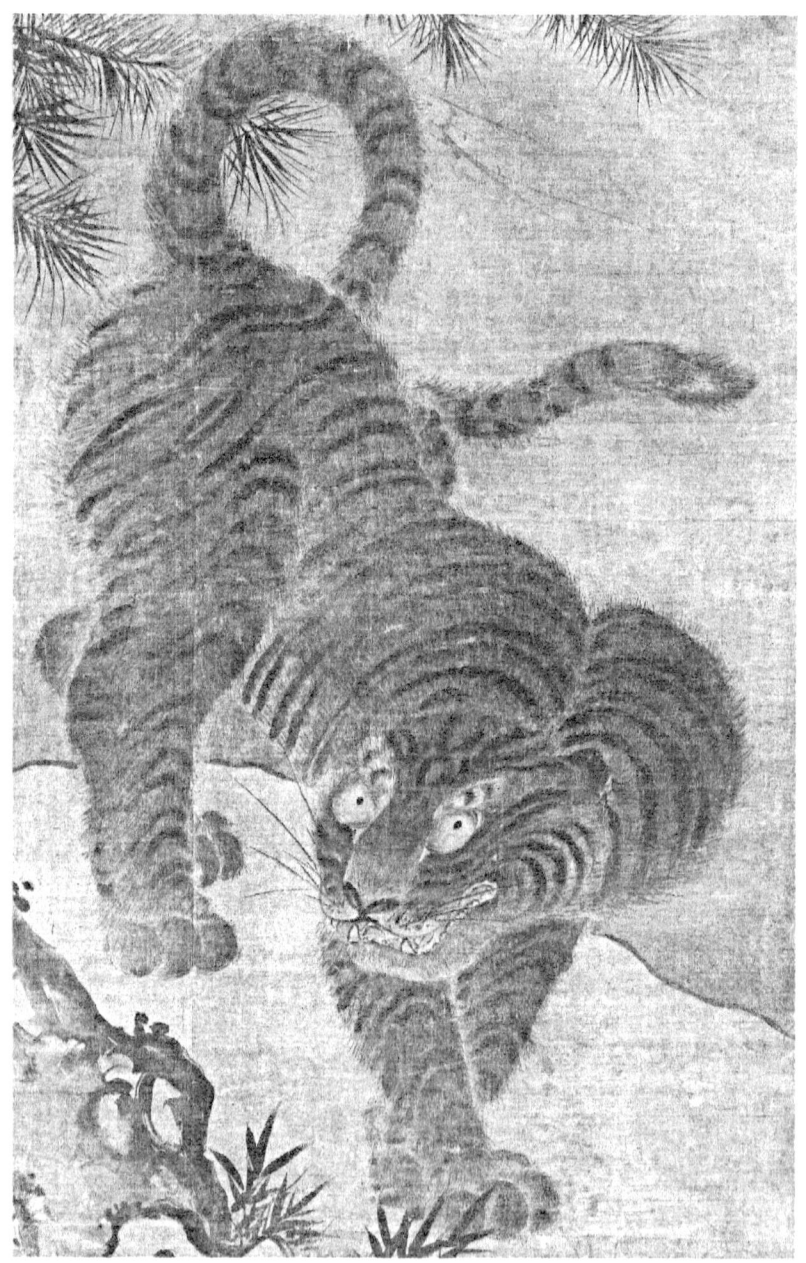

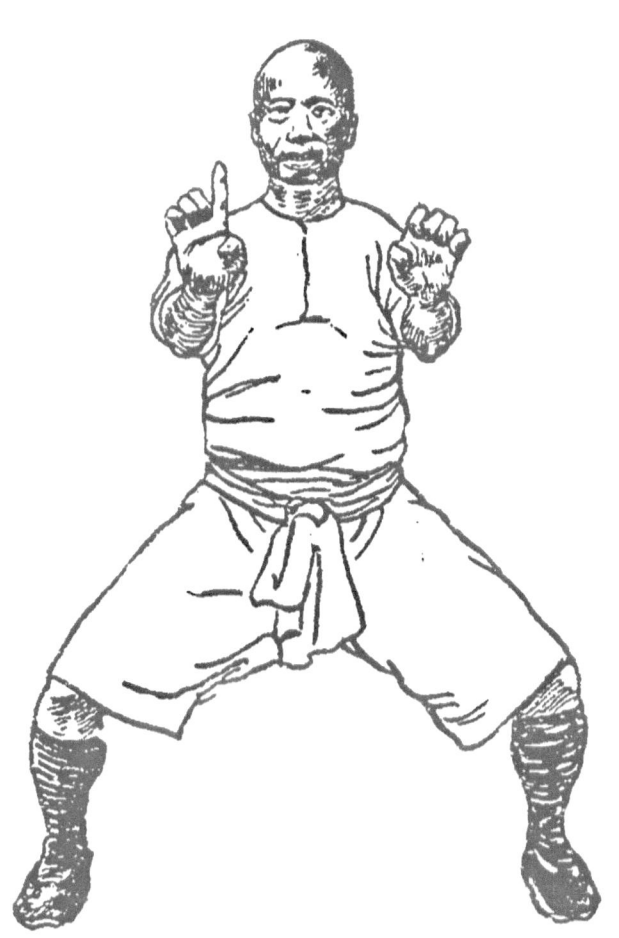

TAMING

the

TIGER

一　合脚離開一寸闊

HE JIAO LI KAI YI CUN KUO (Mandarin)
HAP GEUK LEI HOI JAT CHYUN FUT (Cantonese)

1. Join Your Feet Leaving One Cun[I] Between Them.

Stand straight as if carrying a 1000 Jin[II] weight on the crown of your head. Qi (氣)[III] lowers to Dantian (丹田)[IV], and from there, it spreads to four extremities: the Heart, Feet, Ears, and Eyes. The Heart (Spirit), in conjunction with a Thought (an Intention), reaches the Feet; after it, a state of fullness (with Qi energy) is attained. The Heart feels a presentiment, the Eyes see everything around, and the Ears hear sounds from eight sides.

[I] **Cun** (Cantonese: **Tsun**, 寸) is a traditional Chinese unit of length. Using the traditional (old) standard, one **Cun** measures ≈1.463 in (≈3.715 cm).

[II] **Jin** (Cantonese: **Gan**, 斤) is a traditional Chinese unit for weight. One **Jin** is approximately equal to 1.316 lb (600 grams).

[III] **Qi** (Cantonese: **Hei**, 氣) - in this context, the human internal energy, fundamental "life force" or "vital energy"; the physiological energy of the Microcosm; one of the basic concepts of *Traditional Chinese Medicine* and *Chinese Martial Arts*.

[IV] **Dantian** (Cantonese: **Daantin**, 丹田) - the vital energy center in the human body, according to *Traditional Chinese Medicine*, *Taoist*, and *Buddhist* traditions. Considered the body's powerhouse for storing and cultivating **Qi**. Located in the lower abdomen, about three finger-widths below and two finger-widths behind the navel. It is considered the foundation of rootedness, balance, and breathing. Foundation for physical energy, grounding, and power in martial arts.

Commentaries[I]: The *Shaolin* school of mastering and controlling Breath-*Qi*, known to the Western reader as *Chi Kung* or *Qi Gong*, is an integral part of the *Shaolin* Tradition of Martial Arts. An extract from the book of the Superior of the *Shaolin* monastery *De Chang*[II]:

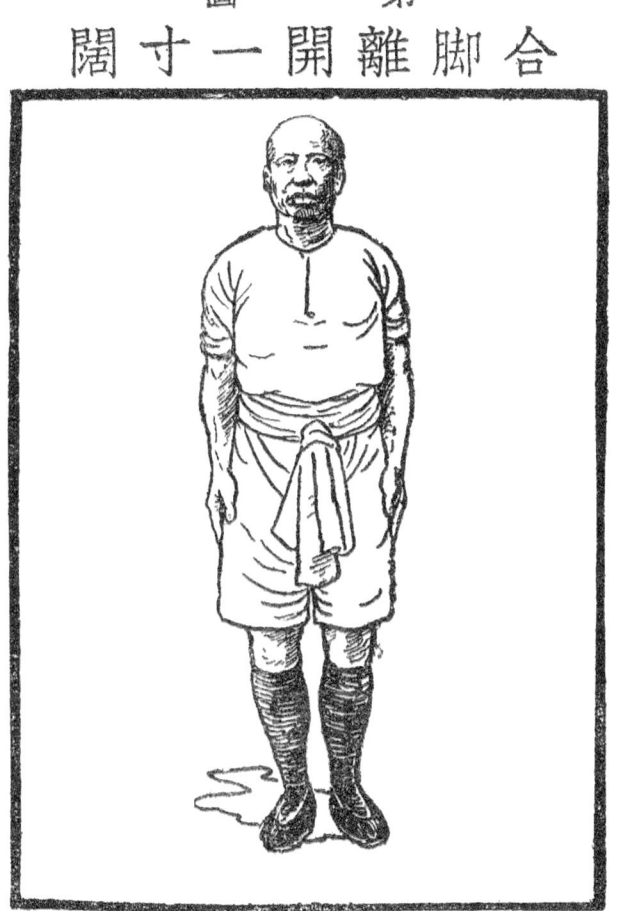

第一圖

合脚離開一寸闊

頭頂千斤氣下丹田由丹田而貫于四肢何爲四肢心
足耳目是爲四肢心則意到足習其標準眼觀四便耳
聽八方

FIG. 1

[I] Commentaries by Andrew Timofeevich (editor of the translation).

[II] De Chang. *Shaolin Qi Gong*. Zhangzhou, 1983.

"The Breath-Qi must unite with the Force-Li, the Mind should keep union with the Heart, the Heart must be in union with the Mind, and the Mind should guide the Breath-Qi. The Breath-Qi moves down and reaches the center of a foot. It also moves up and reaches the top of Kunlun Mountain (i.e., the brain). When you direct Qi with your Mind, you make Qi penetrate the center of the abdominal cavity; in other words, the Breath-Qi is submerged in the Cinnabar Field (Dantian). The law of Cinnabar Field is the base of breathing exercises, and the Force originating from the Cinnabar Field is as strong as the Tiger".

二 兩手揸拳藏在腰

LIANG SHOU ZHA QUAN CANG ZAI YAO (Mandarin)
LEUNG SAU JA KYUN CHONG JOI YIU (Cantonese)

2. Clench Your Fists and Hide them on Your Waist.

Hide your fists near the waist. If your enemy strikes from the left, repulse his blow with your right hand and resort to the grip "Hand Restraining the Tiger"[1]. However, the enemy can make a false movement to conceal his true intentions. Therefore, it is necessary to tell the truth from the false and to react only to a real attack.

Commentaries: This position is the initial position for the next technique and has no independent meaning. Therefore, the

---

[1] *"Hand Restraining the Tiger"*, 伏虎手, *FU HU SHOU* (*Mandarin*), *FOOK FU SAU* (*Cantonese*) - is a technique for gripping an attacking arm of the enemy by the wrist region followed by pressure, from up to down, with the palm to an elbow joint in the direction opposite to its natural curve. This technique and its combat application are described in detail by **Lam Sai Wing** in *Tiger and Crane*, where this method is called *"The Hand of Jin Gang Taming the Tiger"*. *Jin Gang* (*Mandarin*), 金刚, (*Cantonese: Gaam Gong, Sanskrit: Vajrapani*) - a guard of Buddhist temples, an "Iron Warrior" **[index, p. 219]**.

author describes one of the alternatives for fighting, using *"Cutting Palms"* here (see **Fig. 3**). It is especially stressed that you should be on your guard when you conduct a grip, as with a false thrust, the enemy can put you into a dangerous situation.

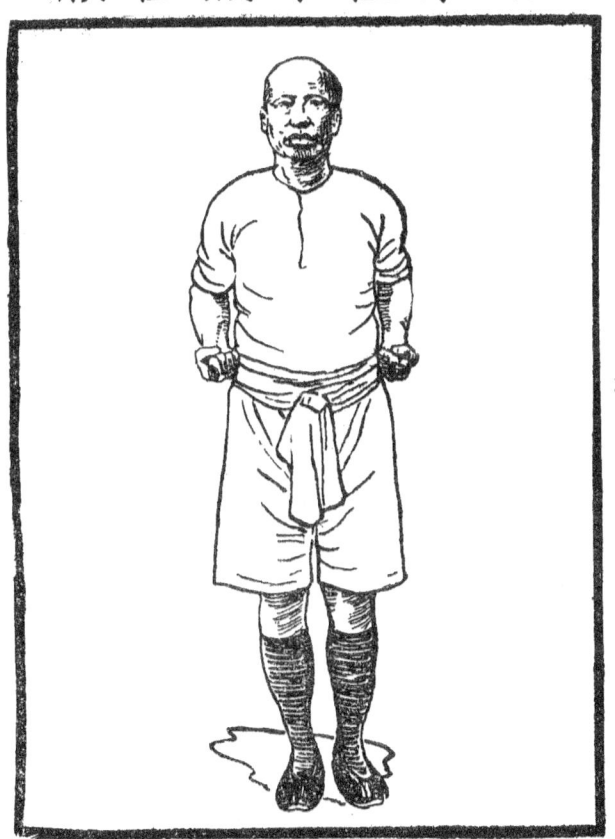

第 二 圖
兩手揸拳藏在腰

藏拳在腰若敵人由左打來則右招右則左招用擒拿
伏虎手虛則虛招實則實擋

FIG. 2

三　抽上胸中一切出

CHOU SHANG XUN ZHONG YI QIE CHU (Mandarin)
CAU SOENG HUNG JUNG JAT CHIT CHEUT (Cantonese)

3. Pull Up Your Hands to the Breast Level and Cut with Palms.

"The cutting palms" means a technique of blocking the opponent's attacking arm from the outside. The hands are in the position "A Pair of Hands like Wings"[I], and the elbows are pressed (to the sides). Step to the side and turn sideways to your opponent. Each time, when dodging an attack and defending the sides, you should "draw rein," that is, to keep the elbows near the sides. Dodge the enemy's blows. Otherwise, you will find ignominious death.

Commentaries: A fighting application of the technique *"Cutting palms"* with displacement from the attack line is described here, whereas, in the routine, this technique is executed from an initial stance with feet close together. A version of passing to the grip *"Hand Restraining the Tiger"* from the position *"The Cutting Palms"* is presented in the description of the previous technique (see **Fig. 2**).

[I] *"A Pair of Hands like Wings"* (雙翅手, *Mandarin:* **SHUANG CHI SHOU**, *Cantonese:* **SEUNG CHI SAU**), an outside block with the edges of palms to deflect a strike away from the defender and across the attacker, **Fig. 3, [see index, p. 222]**.

第三圖
抽上胸中一切出

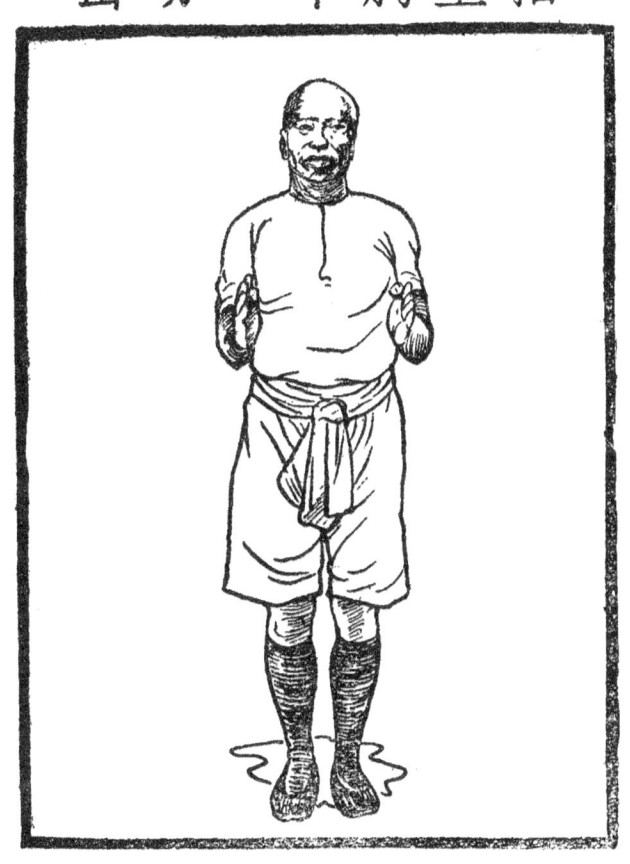

切掌之法即外膊之手法也逢敵人用雙翅手伏我膊
我即用偏身破排逢偏身破排即要拉馬歸後免被伏
死

FIG. 3

四 反手抽拳對膊肩

FAN SHOU CHOU QUAN DUI BO JIAN (Mandarin)
FAAN SAU CAU KYUN DEOI BOK CIN (Cantonese)

4. Turn your Arms, Pull Out Your Fists and Place Your Hands Against Your Shoulders.

The method "Pull out Fists"[1] is executed with both arms. Pull up your clenched fists from your shoulders, then move the elbows aside and do a cutting movement down. This technique can be used to free yourself from the clutch of an opponent who suddenly pounces from behind.

Commentaries: From the position *"The cutting palms"* **(Fig. 3)**, turn your palms upward, clench your hands into fists with force, and slowly and forcefully pull your fists to your shoulders. This phase of conducting the technique is shown in **Fig. 4**. Then, by sending a force to the arms, you jerk fists up with a sharp expiration and lower them to shoulders through the sides. It is a "cutting" movement with elbows from up to down. In the final position, the elbows are pressed to the sides, and the fists are at shoulder level, with the palm centers facing forward.

---

[1] *"Pull Out Fists"* (抽拳, Mandarin: **CHOU QUAN**, Cantonese: **CAU KYUN**) [index, p. 223].

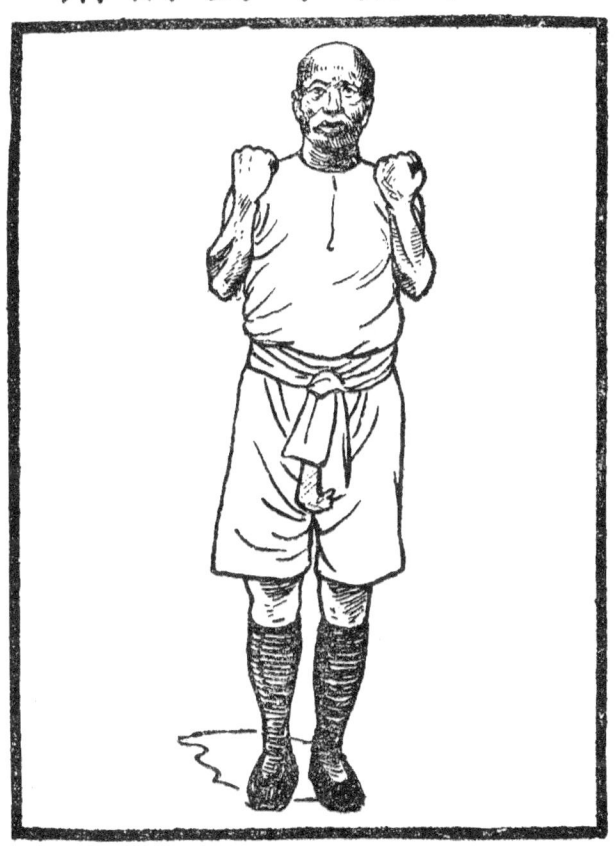

第四圖

反手抽拳對膊肩

抽拳之法雙拳揸實手要抽上若逢敵人在後伏我身
我即將兩手插上一迫可能消之

FIG. 4

五　横迫三株標串掌

HENG PO SAN ZHU BIAO CHUAN ZHANG (Mandarin)
WAANG BIK SAAM JYU BIU CHYUN JEUNG (Cantonese)

5. Push to the Sides Three Times, the Fighting Cock Spreads its Wings, Pierce with Palms.

The "Three Openings"[I] method is designed to train Internal Strength. This is a secret technique of the Hung Gar School. Do the technique "Three Openings" three times. Then execute the "Wing Flaps of the Fighting Cock". Then – "The Fighting Cock spreads its wings," that is a piercing blows with your fingertips asides. The enemy delivers a straight blow at your head. You swiftly use the technique "Do a Mark with a Piercing Hand"[II] to parry the blow and to counterattack.

> **Commentaries:** *"Three openings"* is one of the most important basic techniques of Hung Gar style inherited from the Southern Shaolin. The Shaolin "Treatises on Fighting Arts" say: "It is necessary to pay special attention to the fact that the Mind would guide the Breath-*Qi* and the Breath-*Qi* should act in unity with the physical Force-*Li*. The Breath-*Qi* must strengthen the physical Force-*Li* and the Force-*Li* must guide the Breath-*Qi*". This, in outward appearance, a simple exercise, is aimed at training the said cooperation. The hands are in a position of *"One Finger"* (*JAT ZI*), as shown in **Fig. 13**. The initial position: the palms are on the shoulder level, and the elbows are lowered on the sides. Take a sharp breath in through the mouth and "close"

[I] *"Three Openings"* (三株, Mandarin: *SAN ZHU*, Cantonese: *SAAM ZYU*) **[see index, p. 225].**

[II] *"Do a Mark with a Piercing Hand"* (標串掌, Mandarin: *BIAO CHUAN ZHANG*, Cantonese: *BIU CYUN JEUNG*) - a thrust blow with the ends of fingers of an open palm **[see index, p. 217].**

Qi (strain your stomach and hold breathing), then slowly, with an effort, pull the palms aside on the shoulder level.

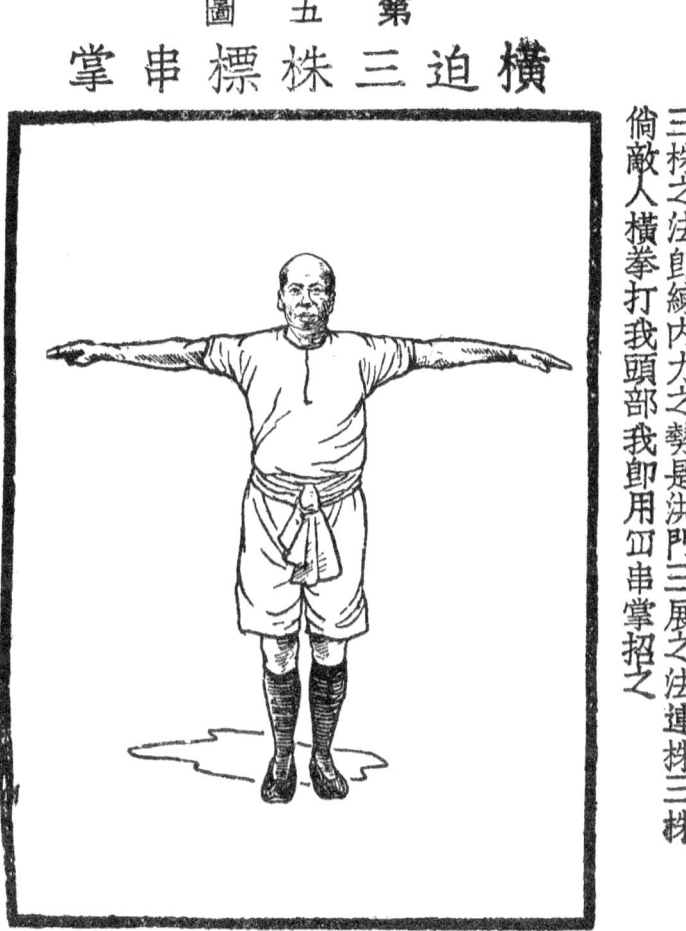

第 五 圖

掌 串 標 株 三 迫 橫

三株之法即練內力之勢是洪門三展之法連株三株
倘敵人橫拳打我頭部我即用皿串掌招之

FIG. 5

The centers of the palms are directed to the sides, and the index fingers are pointing upwards. This movement should be accompanied by a slow, strained exhalation through the nose. Just imagine that you are in a narrow cleft and you are trying to move aside cliffs. This is called *'The Thought leads Qi'*. Then, sharply breathe in and quickly return your arms to the initial position. After the third repetition, lower your open palms along the sides to the waist on both sides with a sharp movement. This is the technique **"Wing Flaps of the**

Fighting Cock". Then, without stopping, strike a piercing blows to the sides with the tips of your fingers, as shown in **Fig. 5**. This is the technique *"Fighting Cock Spreads its Wings".*

六　沉睜一定指撐天

CHEN ZHENG YI DING ZHI CHENG TIAN (Mandarin)
CAM ZAANG JAT DING ZI CAANG TIN (Cantonese)

6. Submerge Your Elbows and Support the Sky with Your Fingers.

Four of your fingers support the sky, and the elbows are "submerged."[I] This is one of the secret methods of the Hung Gar style, known as "The Iron Hand of the Buddhist Tutor."[II] If you want to master the power at your fingertips, practice the method "Four Fingers Support the Sky."[III]

Commentaries: This position has no direct practical use. However, like the technique *"Three openings,"* it is part of the treasury of Hard *Qi Gong* of *Hung Gar* style methods. It is

---

[I] It means the following stance: the hands are put aside at shoulder level; the arms are slightly bent; the elbows are faced down and lowered somewhat.

[II] *"The Iron Hand of the Buddhist Tutor"* (鉄臂禪師, Mandarin: *ZHI BI CHAN SHI*, Cantonese: *TIT BEI SIM SI*) - a set of special exercises for developing the strength of the hands and fingers, practiced in the *Southern Shaolin* styles. Mastering these methods enables one to deliver powerful blows with a "tiger paw" and execute effective grabs **[index, p. 220]**.

[III] *"Four Fingers Support the Sky"* (四指撐天, Mandarin: *SI ZHI CHENG TIAN*, Cantonese: *SEI ZI CAANG TIN*) - four of your fingers are completely straight and spread wide with effort, the thumb is perpendicular to the palm plane and directed forward. Your wrists are bent toward the outer side of your forearms. You should feel some tension in your wrists, thumbs, and fingers. This is one of the basic exercises for strengthening hands, fingers and forearms **[index, p. 218]**.

also the heritage of the *Kung Fu* School of Southern *Shaolin*. An obligatory condition of its execution is that four fingers are completely straightened and spread apart with force, and the thumb is perpendicular to the plane of the palm. This exercise develops all sinews of the forearm and strengthens fingers. The Tiger style of the Southern *Shaolin*, which served as a base for creating this form (*TAO LU*) and the formation of *Hung Gar* as a whole, includes many blows with "tiger's claws", fingers, and grips. Therefore, the strengthening of fingertips is of great importance here.

第 六 圖

天 撐 指 定 一 胂 沉

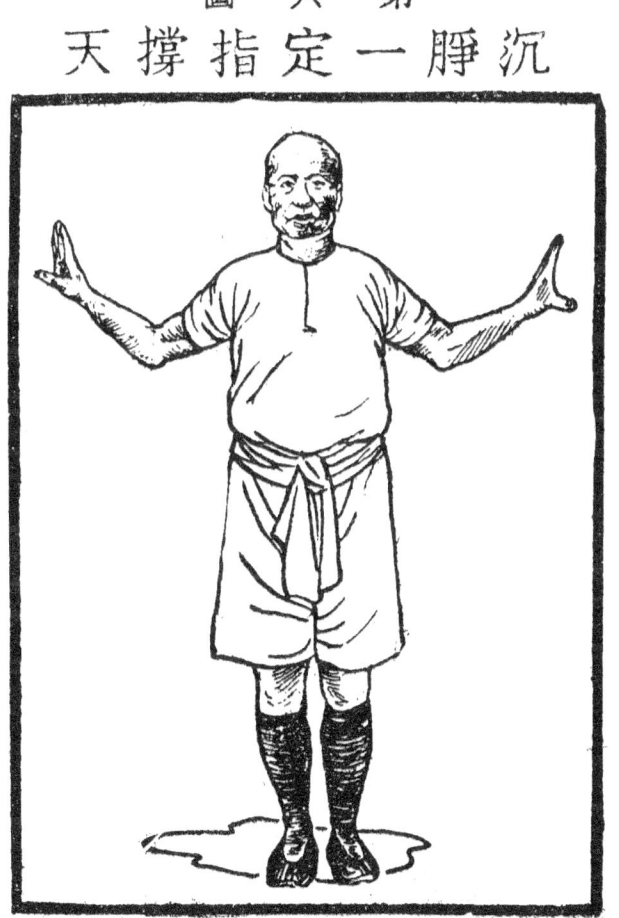

法 四指撐天天上天沉胂對膊是真言莫話洪拳無妙法
鐵臂禪師也是言欲用指尾之力必要練四指撐天之

FIG. 6

七 右手揸拳左用掌

YOU SHOU ZHA QUAN ZUO YONG ZHANG (Mandarin)
JAU SAU ZAA KYUN JO YUNG JEUNG (Cantonese)

7. Clench Your Right Hand into Fist, use Your Left Palm.

If the enemy delivers a punch at the middle part of your torso, you immediately use "A Hand Like a Wing"[I] method, bounce his blow, and punch with your fist. Regardless of the technique or style the attacking enemy uses, you immediately apply the "The Hungry Tiger catches the Sheep"[II] technique and defeat him.

Commentaries: The positions in **Fig. 7** and **Fig. 8** are two phases of one technique. **Fig. 7** shows the first phase: a block with a hand in the shape of a wing (翅手, *CHI SAU*) and the preparation for a punch. **Fig. 8** shows the second phase: a punch with the right fist and the preparation to grip an enemy's arm with your left hand. The text to **Fig. 7** describes one of the options for further actions from the position shown in **Fig. 8**: if the opponent blocks your strike with his left forearm, pass to execute the technique *"The Hungry Tiger Catches the Sheep."*

[I] *"A Hand Like a Wing"* (翅手, Mandarin: *CHI SHOU*, Cantonese: *CHI SAU*) an outside block with the edge of the palm to deflect a strike away from the defender and across the attacker **(Fig. 3) [see index, p. 219]**.

[II] *"The Hungry Tiger Catches the Sheep"* (餓虎擒羊, Mandarin: *E HU QIN YANG*, Cantonese: *NGO FU KAM YEUNG*) means to grip an enemy's arm in the wrist region with one hand and sharply pull to yourself and down. Simultaneously, with the forearm of another arm, using body weight, press on the elbow of the gripped hand in the direction opposite its natural curve. This technique is described in detail by **Lam Sai Wing** in *Tiger and Crane* **[index, p. 220]**.

右手揸拳左拳用掌

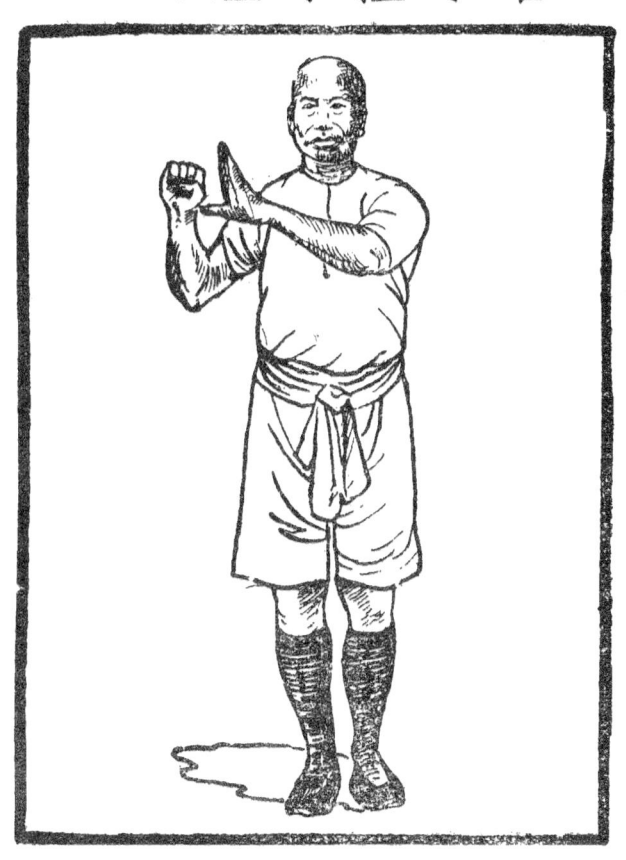

逢敵人中拳打我我即用翅手翅他胮部連環一拳打他無論敵人用何拳勢攻我我即用餓虎擒羊之法以消之

FIG. 7

八　吊脚收胸見禮謙

DIAO JIAO SHOU XUN JIAN LI QIAN (Mandarin)
DIU GEUK SAU HYUN GIN LAI HIM (Cantonese)

8. Suspend Your Foot, Pull in Your Breast[I], Perform the Greeting Ceremony.

When you meet a follower of another school of Martial Arts, first of all, you should exercise a greeting ceremony. If the enemy suddenly attacks you with his fist at the middle part of your torso, immediately use the technique "A Hand Like a Wing"[II]. This movement, without any stop, transforms into the method "Lock the Iron Gate with a Bolt Weighing 1000 Jins."[III]

Commentaries: Here, a characteristic feature of traditional martial arts is emphasized: in any situation, one must be on guard and not allow oneself to be taken by surprise. Even at the moment of a greeting, one should be ready to repel a sudden

---

[I] Requirements to the stance **(Fig. 8)**: The shoulders are slightly advanced, the chest is slightly drawn inward ("empty"), the stomach is "filled" and tensed. Because of it, **Qi** moves down and concentrates in **Dantian**. The center of your body weight is in a lower position, the position is stable, and your attention is concentrated. If the breast is "filled," i.e., thrust out, then **Qi** is rushing up, the position is not stable, and it is difficult to achieve concentration.

[II] **A Hand Like a Wing"** (翅手, Mandarin: **CHI SHOU**, Cantonese: **CHI SAU**) - an outside block with the edge of the palm to deflect a strike away from the defender and across the attacker **[see index, p. 219]**.

[III] **"Lock the Iron Gate with a Bolt Weighing 1000 Jin"** (鐵門閂槌千斤, Mandarin: **TIE MEN SHUAN CHUI QIAN JIN**, Cantonese: - **TIT MUN SAAN CHEUI CIN GAN**) - a technique that has various applications, which are described later in this book (see **Fig. 82**), as well as in Lam Sai Wing's book **"Tiger and Crane"**. In this case, it refers to a simultaneous punch with both fists, from the bottom up, with an upward movement, aimed at the opponent's stomach and neck (or chin). **Jin** (Cantonese: **Gan**, 斤) is a traditional Chinese unit for weight. One **Jin** is approximately equal to 1.316 lb (600 grams) **[see index, p. 221]**.

attack. Further is considered an alternative way of action from the position in **Fig. 8**. If the enemy beats off your punch with his forearm from down to up, immediately pass to the technique *"Lock the Iron Gate with a Bolt Weighing 1000 Jin"*: catch the blocking arm of the enemy with your left hand and sharply pull it down and to yourself. The next moment, deliver a simultaneous blow with two fists, from bottom to top, with an upward movement, to the opponent's stomach and neck (or chin).

第 八 圖

吊 脚 收 胸 見 禮 謙

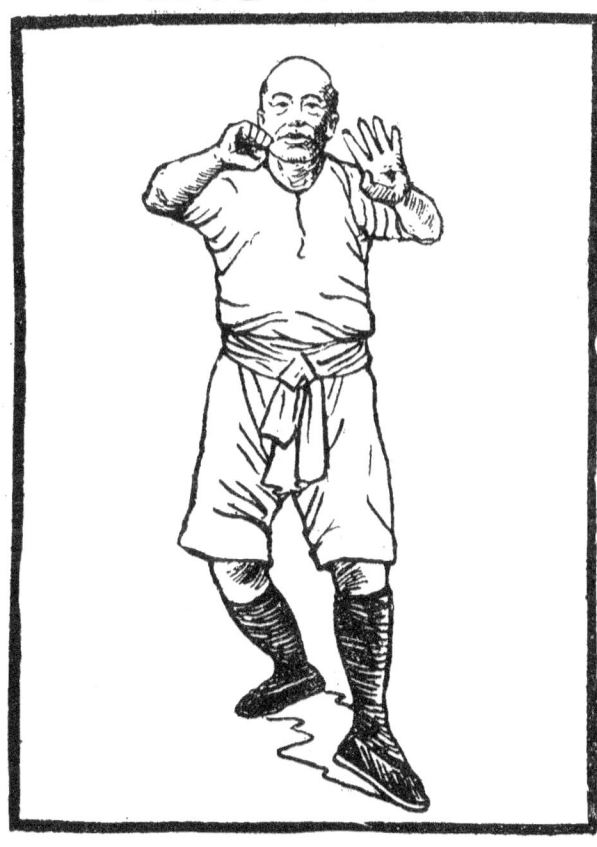

逢拳術家必先以禮相見倘敵人一拳由中打來我即用□翅手服之連轉鉄門門千斤墜之法

FIG. 8

九 扭手收拳歸原位

NIU SHOU SHOU QUAN GUI YUAN WEI (Mandarin)
NAU SAU SAU KYUN GWAI YUN WAI (Cantonese)

9. Turn your Hands, Bring Together Your Fists, Return to the Initial Position.

Pull your fists to your waist, and Qi moves into Dantian. The enemy uses the method "Palms like Butterflies."[I] I also use the "Palms like Butterflies" for a counterattack. If the enemy is stronger than I am and suppresses my attack by force, I immediately proceed to the technique "Turn and Divide, Penetrate with Hands"[II] and deliver a blow.

Commentaries: If the enemy attacks with the ***"Palms like butterflies"*** (蝶掌, ***DIP JEUNG***), you also meet him with your ***"Palms like butterflies"*** to deflect his blows outside. But the enemy, trying to "entangle" your arms and to engage you in a close fight, exerts pressure on your arms from outside to inside. In this case, it is necessary to "draw" a circle with your hands before your chest, placing your arms outside the enemy's arms and following their movement in the previous direction. Thus, you use enemy's force against him. Then you strike at the gap in his defense, which has appeared. All movements are done at once, as the outcome of a close fight is determined in a few seconds.

[I] ***"Palms like Butterflies"*** (蝶掌, Mandarin: ***DIE ZHANG***, Cantonese: ***DIP JEUNG***) - circular block with both palms in the frontal plane, followed by a simultaneous blow with open palms at two levels, the fingers of the upper palm are directed upwards, the fingers of the lower palm are directed downwards **(Figs. 52, 63, 66, 89)**, [see index, p. 223].

[II] ***"Turn and Divide, Penetrate with Hands"*** (轉分漏手, Mandarin: ***ZHUAN FEN LOU SHOU***, Cantonese: ***JYUN FAN LAU SAU***) - see commentaries above **[see index, p. 226]**.

扭手收拳歸原位

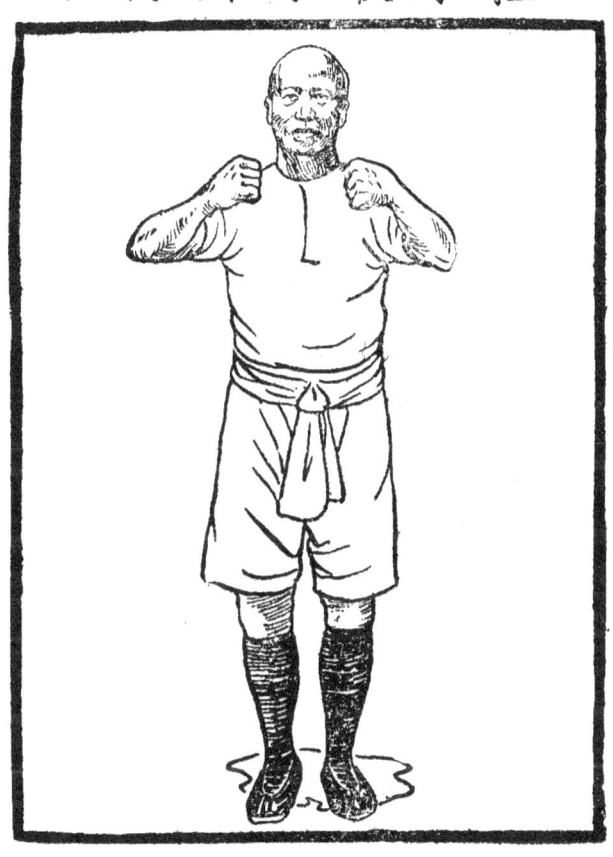

收拳腰部氣運丹田敵人一蝶掌打來我亦用蝶掌招
之倘他力大伏我我即轉分漏手法破之

FIG. 9

十　脚挣開馬落四平
JIAO ZHENG KAI MA LUO SEI PING (Mandarin)
GEUK ZAANG HOI MAA LOK SEI PING (Cantonese)

10. Stand on Your Feet Apart and Take a Stable Stance *SEI PING MAA.*

In the SEI PING MAA[I] Stance, the ends of your feet are placed exactly under your knees, the head (neck) is kept vertically, and the waist is "submerged" (lowered). Those are essential things in the SEI PING MAA Stance. The enemy attacks using the technique of "Uninterrupted Punches like Rockets."[II] Submerge into the stable SEI PING MAA Stance and use "The Piercing Bridge"[III] to repulse his attack.

Commentaries: Training of the stance **SEI PING MA** ("Horse Stance") is one of the basic exercises in the style of *Hung Gar*. It was believed earlier that if a learner cannot stand in this stance for at least twenty minutes, there is no sense in teaching him fighting methods. Masters could stand in the **SEI**

_____

[I] **"Horse Riding Stance"** (四平馬, Mandarin: **SEI PING MA**, Cantonese: **SEI PING MAA**) – literally: **"Four Levels Horse Stance"**, also known as the **"Horse Stance"** (馬步, **MA BU**) **(Fig. 10)**, **[see index, p. 220]**.

[II] **"Uninterrupted Punches like Rockets"** or **"Fists like Rockets Strike one after another"** (火箭連環拳, Mandarin: **HUO JIAN LIAN HUAN QUAN**, Cantonese: **FO JIN LIN WAAN KYUN**) - a rapid succession of punches, following each other without a break, like rain drumming on a roof **[see index, p. 227]**.

[III] **"The Piercing Bridge"** (穿橋, Mandarin: **CHUN QIAO**, Cantonese: **CHYUN KIU**) – One of the 12 basic techniques (十二支橋, **"12 Bridges"**, **Sahp Yih Ji Kiu**) of the **Hung Gar** style. The hand is in the position shown in **Fig. 13**. The arm is slightly bent at the elbow and stretched forward, and the elbow is turned down and slightly lowered **[index, p. 223]**. See also Lam Sai Wing, **Iron Thread. Southern Shaolin Hung Gar Kung Fu Classics Series** (2008).

PING MA stance for an hour or more. Here is one of the ways to use a low stance in a fight.

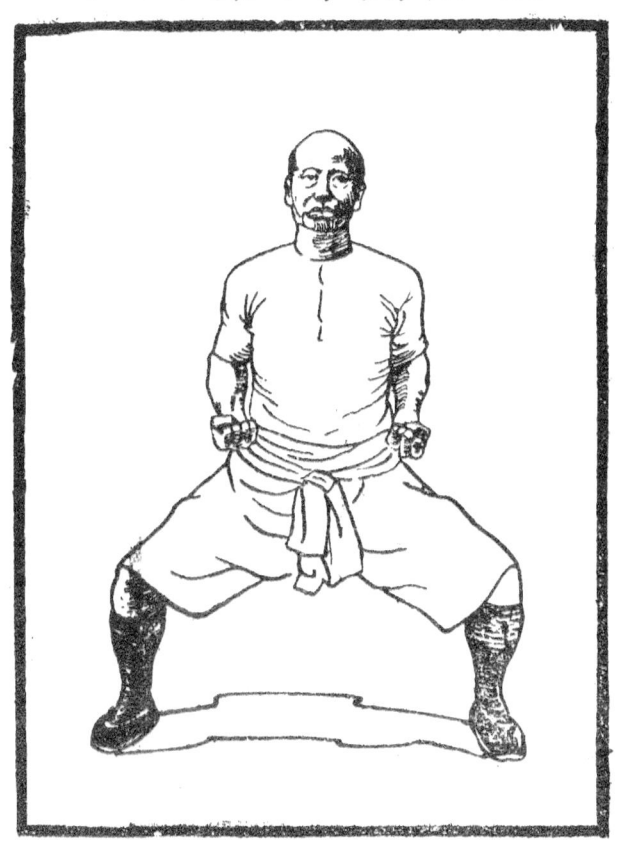

第十圖
脚脛開馬落四平

遵四平馬以脚尖對正膝頭插腰落馬乃合若敵人用火箭連環拳攻我卽用退馬穿橋以消之

FIG. 10

十一　抽拳在胸雙切膀

CHOU QUAN ZAI XUN SHUANG QIE BANG (Mandarin)
CAU KYUN JOI HUNG SEUNG CHIT BONG (Cantonese)

11. Raise Your Fists in Front of Your Breast and Cut with a Pair of Wings[I].

Raise your fists up to the central part of the breast. The enemy attacks you with a punch at the middle level. Immediately "cut" with the edges of your palm moving from up to down. If the enemy continues his attack with blows from the left, parry with your left arm; if he attacks from the right, use your right arm. At the same time as the block, strike with the edge of the palm of your other hand. This technique is called the "Paired Work of 1000 Characters"[II].

Commentaries: The Chinese symbol (character) **"thousand"** (千) consists of two crossed lines - vertical and horizontal. When you execute the method *"Paired Work of 1000 Characters"*, one arm moves from down to upward with a blocking movement, which corresponds to the vertical line of the character; the other arm delivers a straight front blow (or blocking), which corresponds to its horizontal line. Not to be confused with the *"Hand of 1000 Characters"* technique, which appears later in the text. The *"Hand of 1000 Characters"* is a wide range of blows and blocking with the arm (forearm), both from the inside out and the outside in, at

---

[I] *"Cutting with Wings"* (切膀, Mandarin: *QIE BANG*, Cantonese: *CHIT BONG*) – blocking with the outer sides of the forearms with the edges of the palm from top to bottom (**Figs. 11, 47**), **[index, p. 216]**.

[II] *"Paired Work of 1000 Characters"* (雙工千字, Mandarin: *SHUANG GONG QIAN ZI*, Cantonese: *SEUNG GUNG CHIN JI*) - Simultaneous action with both arms: one arm blocks the opponent's strike at the top level with a bottom-up movement, the other hand blocks (or strikes) at the middle level with a horizontal movement **[see index, p. 222]**.

different angles to the line of attack. See also: **Lam Sai Wing,** *Tiger and Crane,* **Fig. 50.**

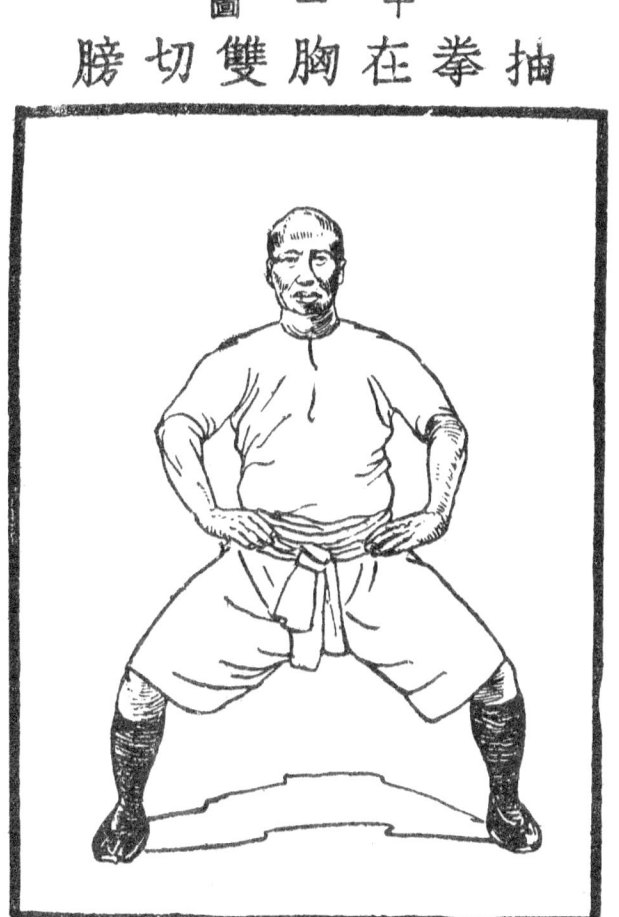

圖 一 十
膀切雙胸在拳抽

將拳抽上胸中倫敵人用中拳打入我即將切膀手招
之倫他再用拳打來左即左招右即右擋或用雙工千
字破之

FIG. 11

十二　合掌分開定金橋

HE ZHANG FEN KAI DING JIN QIAO (Mandarin)
HAP JEUNG FAN HOI DING GAM KIU (Cantonese)

12. Close Your Palms and Part Them to the Position "Stable Gold Bridge".

If the enemy attacks with the method "Palms like Butterflies"[I], I parry it with the technique "Stable Gold Bridge"[II]. If the enemy proceeds to the technique "The Hand Breaking a Line"[III], I immediately "draw the rein", retreat back and use the leg technique "Three-Star Hook Spring Leg"[IV].

Commentaries: Fig. 12 shows the position of the *"Stable Gold Bridge"* (定金橋): the arms are extended forward at chest level, parallel to each other, but not fully straightened; elbows pointing down; four of your fingers are completely straight and spread wide with effort, the thumb is perpendicular to the palm plane and directed forward. Your wrists are bent toward the outer side of your forearms. You should feel some

---

[I] *"Palms like Butterflies"* (蝶掌, Mandarin: *DIE ZHANG*, Cantonese: *DIP JEUNG*) [see index, p. 223].

[II] *"Stable Gold Bridge"* (定金橋, Mandarin: *DING JIN QIAO*, Cantonese: *DING GAM KIU*) - see commentaries above **(Figs. 12, 48, pp. 50, 122) [see index, p. 224]**.

[III] *"The Hand Breaking a Line"* (破排手, Mandarin: *PO PAI SHOU*, Cantonese: *PO PAI SAU*) - Circle and push blocking movements with palms and forearms, which can be performed in a vertical, horizontal, or diagonal direction **[see index, p. 218]**.

[IV] *"Three-Star Hook Spring Leg"* (三星鉤彈腳, Mandarin: *SAN XING ZHU TAN JIAO*, Cantonese: *SAAM SING KAU TAAN GEUK*) - a low sweeping kick with the shin (lower shinbone), hooking and sweeping of the front-standing leg of the enemy, followed by a kick to the knee or ankle of his supporting leg or a reverse leg sweep **[see index, p. 226]**.

tension in your wrists and thumbs. This is one of the basic exercises for strengthening the forearms. See also Lam Sai Wing, ***Iron Thread. Southern Shaolin Hung Gar Kung Fu Classics Series*** (2008).

The literal translation of **PO PAI SAU** means ***"The Hand Breaking a Line."*** If the enemy tries to "entangle" your arms and engage you in a close fight, it is necessary to step back and use the technique of ***"Three-Star Hook Spring Leg".***

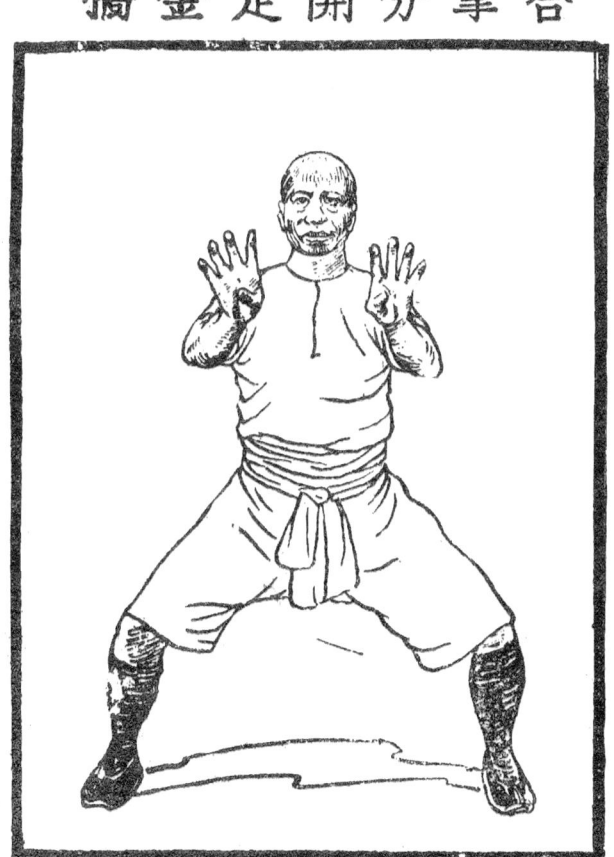

圖 二 十

合掌分開定金橋

倘敵人用蝶掌打來我即用定金橋招之他用破排手
伏我我即拉馬歸後連轉三星扚彈脚法

FIG. 12

十三 一指三株抛脺手

YI ZHI SAN ZHU PAO ZHENG SHOU (Mandarin)
JAT ZI SAAM ZYU PAAU ZAANG SAU (Cantonese)

13. Throw One Finger with Tense Arms Three Times.

The technique "Three Openings" (三展)[1] in the style of Hung Family (洪家) includes three movements that follow one after another. This method is used for the development of an internal force and this force is like a thunder. Besides, this method of the Pugilistic Arts can cure indigestion.

Commentaries: The method of execution of the technique *"Three openings"* is explained in the commentaries to **Fig. 5**. The only difference is that in this case *"Three openings"* is executed in the "Horse Stance" (**Fig. 13**) and it is necessary to "press" with palms in the frontal direction.

---

[1] *"Three Openings"* (三株, Mandarin: **SAN ZHU**, Cantonese: **SAAM ZYU**) is one of the most important basic techniques of **Hung Gar** style inherited from the *Southern Shaolin*. The *Shaolin "Treatises on Fighting Arts"* say: *"It is necessary to pay special attention to the fact that the Mind would guide the Breath-Qi and the Breath-Qi should act in unity with the physical Force-Li. The Breath-Qi must strengthen the physical Force-Li and the Force-Li must guide the Breath-Qi"*. This, in outward appearance, a simple exercise, is aimed at training the said cooperation. The hands are in a position of *"One Finger"* (**JAT ZI**), as shown in **Fig. 13**. The initial position: the palms are on the shoulder level, and the elbows are lowered on the sides. Take a sharp breath in through the mouth and "close" *Qi* (strain your stomach and hold breathing), then slowly, with an effort, pull the palms aside on the shoulder level **[index, p. 225]**.

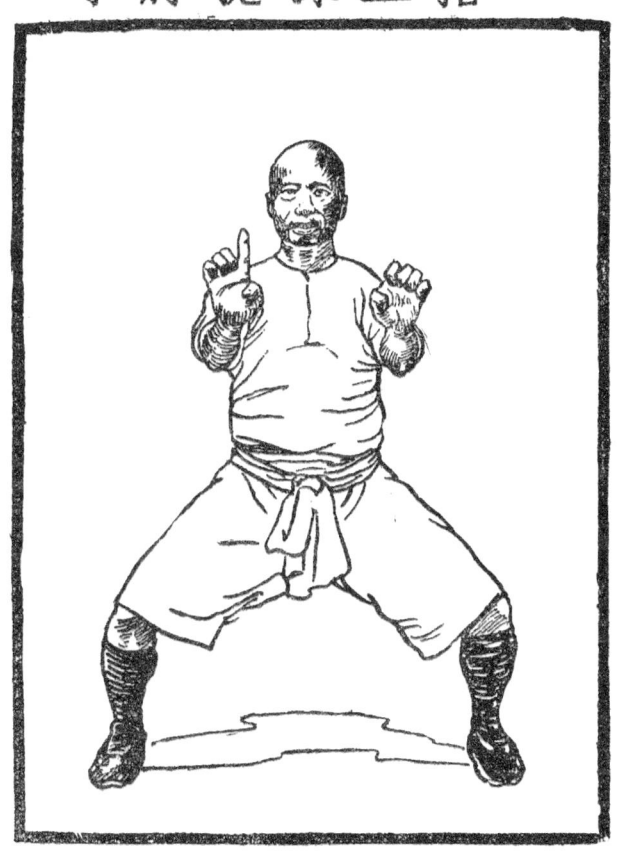

十三圖
手睜拋株三指一

洪家三展之法連株三株用內力震出可助消化食而
不化必要運動拳術消化之

FIG. 13

十四　連拋三次有三勻

LIAN PAO SAN CI YOU SAN YUN (Mandarin)
LIN PAAU SAAM CHI JAU SAAM WAN (Cantonese)

14. To Powder Yourself Three Times and to Deliver Three Blows in Succession.

"To meet with elbows" means to remove the enemy's elbow with your elbow - that is, without fail! If the enemy attacks with a lateral elbow, you parry it with your straight one; if he attacks with a straight elbow, you also parry it with your straight one; if with a raising elbow, you should move your head aside. If the enemy proceeds to an attack with his head, parry it with your leg by striking with your knee on his head. This is the truth of the Pugilistic Art.

Commentaries: After the execution of **"Three openings"**, the hands are transformed from the position of **"Single finger"** to **"Tiger's claws"** and moved to the ears, as shown in **Fig. 14**. The movement is fast, as if throwing handfuls of powder to your face. The meaning of this movement is to protect yourself against an enemy's attack on your head. Then, lower **"The Tiger's claws"** to your waist. This is to parry a blow at your abdomen or your breast. The mode of this movement is as if throwing something: the movement is fast and sharp. After that, deliver a double blow on the enemy's breast with **"Tiger's claws"**. This series of three movements is repeated three times.

十四圖
連拋三次有三勾

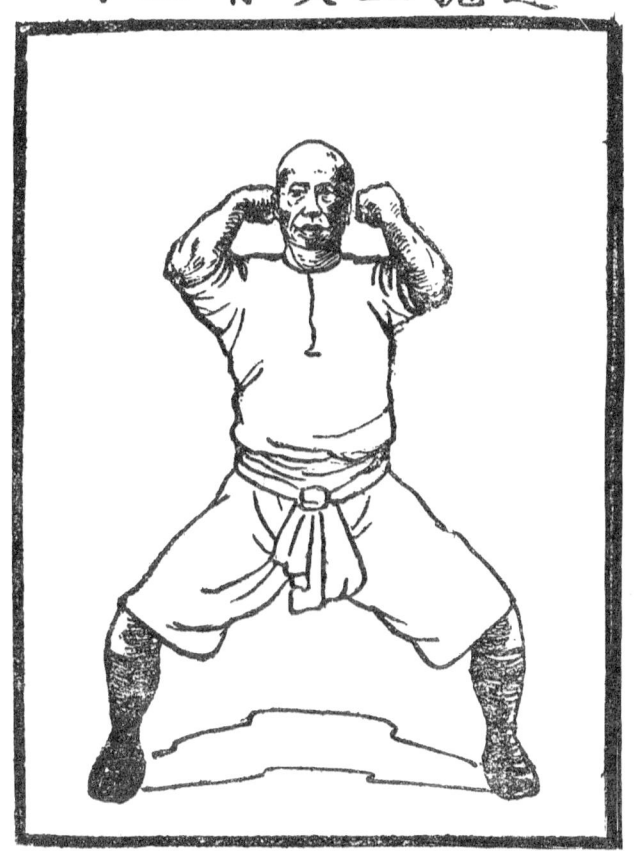

進肨必要以肨消肨橫肨來直肨送直肨來橫肨消頭
來用頭消脚來用脚破此乃拳術之眞理也

FIG. 14

十五 四拋標串撐天指

SI PAO BIAO CHUAN CHENG TIAN ZHI (Mandarin)
SEI PAAU BIU CYUN CAANG TIN ZI (Cantonese)

15. Throw for the Fourth Time, Pierce with Your Fingers, Support the Sky with Your Fingers.

If the enemy attacks my breast or my stomach with a fist, I immediately use the technique "Do a Mark with a Piercing Hand"[I] and pierce his heart and kidneys. If the enemy escapes my blow and tries to hold my hand, I eliminate his clench and suppress him with a method called "The Hand Breaking a Line"[II].

Commentaries: After performing the previous technique three times, "powder" yourself a fourth time (**Fig. 14**), then move your hands to your waist and, without stopping, deliver a double piercing blow forward, at chest level, with the fingertips of both hands. Then, quickly lower your arms, slightly bent at the elbows, to the solar plexus level with your fingers straightened and pointing upward (**Fig. 15**).

[I] *"Do a Mark with a Piercing Hand"* (標串手, Mandarin: ***BIAO CHUAN SHOU***, Cantonese: ***BIU CYUN SAU***) - a thrusting blow with the ends of fingers of an open palm [index, p. 217].

[II] *"The Hand Breaking a Line"* (破排手, Mandarin: ***PO PAI SHOU***, Cantonese: ***PO PAI SAU***) - circle and push blocking movements with palms and forearms, which can be performed in a vertical, horizontal, or diagonal direction [index, p. 218].

十五圖
四拋標串撐天指

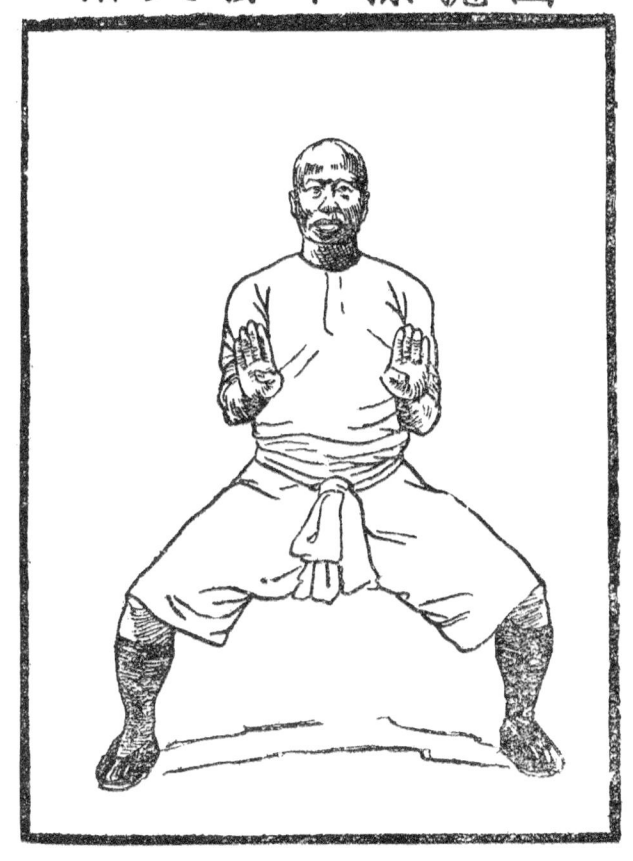

倘敵人一拳向中部打來我即用標串手寫他心脅即連消帶打之法他招我我即用班中破排手法伏之

FIG. 15

十六　雙抽雙割一揸分

SHUANG CHOU SHUANG GE YI ZHA FEN (Mandarin)
SEUNG CAU SEUNG GOT JAT ZA FAN (Cantonese)

16. Both Pull Out and Both Cut, Grasp and Bring Apart.

Cross your forearms before your breast, clench your hands into fists, continuously move down and bring them apart in front of the lower stomach to do the technique "Dividing the Gold Bridge"[I]. If the enemy delivers you a blow, cross your hands against the center of your breast and move ahead in the stance MA[II], beat off the attacking arm of the enemy, and punch without any delay.

Commentaries: *"Dividing the Gold Bridge"* is a movement as if tearing some cloth, the effort is burst-like, the blow (or block) is delivered with the back of your fist or with your forearm **(Fig. 16)**.

[I] *"Dividing the Gold Bridge"* (分金橋, Mandarin: *FEN JIN QIAO*, Cantonese: *FAN GAM KIU*) - a movement as if tearing some cloth, the effort is burst-like, the blow is delivered with the back of your fist or with your forearm **[see index, p. 217]**.

[II] *"Horse Riding Stance"* (四平馬, Mandarin: *SEI PING MA*, Cantonese: *SEI PING MAA*) – literally: *"Four Levels Horse Stance"*, also known as the *"Horse Stance"* (馬步, *MA BU*) **(Fig. 10)**, [index, p. 220].

十 六 圖
分揸一割雙抽雙

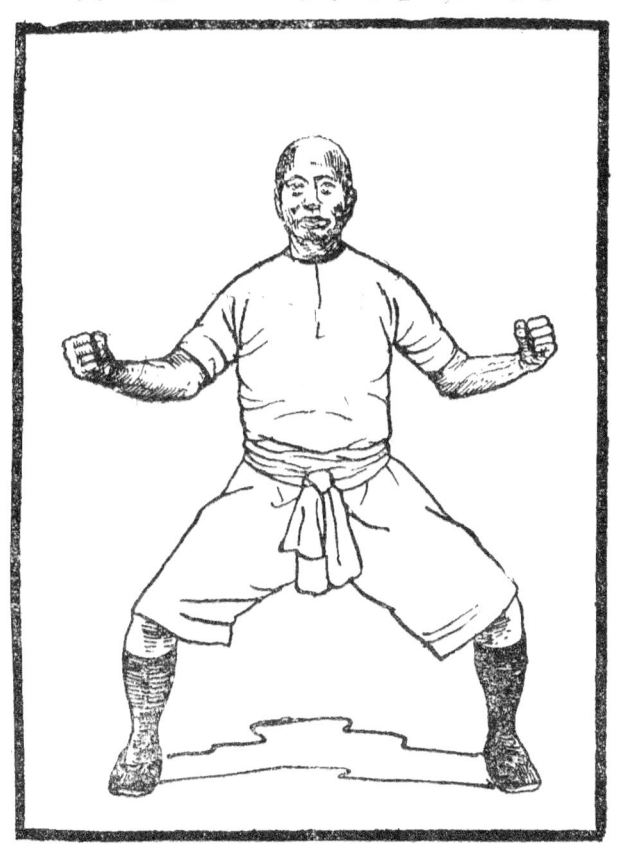

逢雙膀手揸拳在臍下連環一分即分金橋之法倘敵
人打來我即用膊手對他心胸進馬一分即掛打拳法
連消帶打

FIG. 16

十七　出左吊右拉歸後

CHU ZUO DIAO YOU LA GUI HOU (Mandarin)
CHEUT JO DIU JAU LAAI GWAI HAU (Cantonese)

17. Go Out to the Left, Hang on the Right, Draw the Rein, and Come Back.

Step with your left foot, "draw the rein," come back, turn your torso to the right, and raise your right foot. If the enemy attacks with a kick, I immediately beat off his blow with my raised foot.

Commentaries: From the previous position **(Fig.16)**, your left foot steps to the left. You turn the body to the right and take the stance shown in **Fig. 17**. Then, your right foot steps back. You take the position shown in **Fig. 18** without interrupting movement. All movements are done fast and continuously without pausing.

十七圖

出左吊右拉歸後

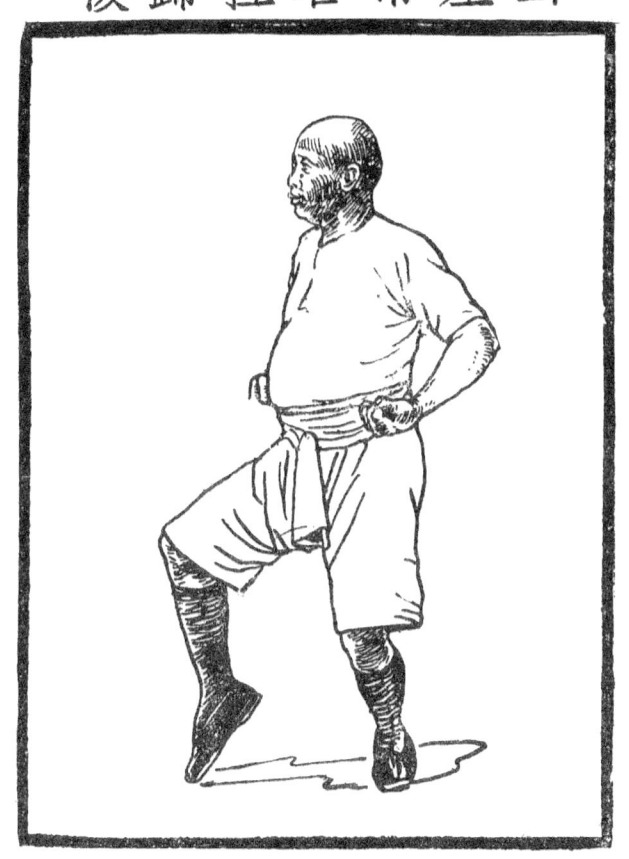

用左脚一出拉馬歸後身向右將脚一起倘敵人用脚打來我即用脚消之即脚上起脚之法

FIG. 17

十八　鏟脚四平八分馬

CHAN JIAO SEI PING BA FEN MA (Mandarin)
CHAN GEUK SEI PING BAAT FAN MAA (Cantonese)

18. A Foot Like a Spade, Lower Yourself to the Posture SEI PING BA FEN MA.

My foot "cuts" like a spade. I lower myself to the stance SEI PING BAAT FAN MAA[I]. If the enemy punches me at the middle level from behind, I immediately turn my feet to the stance JI NG MAA[II] and block his attack with the DAAN BONG SAU[III].

Commentaries: After parrying your enemy's kick with your right foot, you deliver a side kick with the edge of your foot on the knee of his supporting leg without stopping the movement. Then, you lower yourself to the position of ***"Stable Horse Riding Stance"*** (Fig. 10).

Note: Here and further, in some cases, pictures do not fully correspond with the text. Sometimes, the text, to a greater extent, belongs to further figures or describes actions that are

---

[I] *"Stable Horse Riding Stance"* (四平八分馬, Mandarin: ***SEI PING BA FEN MA***, Cantonese: ***SEI PING BAAT FAN MAA***) – literally: ***"Four Levels Eight Parts Horse Stance"*** - lower *"Horse Stance"*, i.e., the feet are widespread, the center of gravity is situated low **(Fig. 10) [see index, p. 225]**.

[II] ***JI NG MAA*** (子午馬, Mandarin: ***ZI WU MA***, Cantonese: ***JI NG MAA***) - known in the modern *WUSHU* as the stance **"Bow and Arrow" (Fig. 19)**. The term **"MA"** is used in the meaning "a stance" here **[see index, p. 220]**.

[III] ***"Single Arm like a Wing"*** (單膀手, Mandarin: ***DAN BANG SHOU***, Cantonese: ***DAAN BONG SAU***) - a forearm block **[see index, p. 224]**.

not illustrated. However, it reflects the original text, and we did not think it appropriate to change anything.

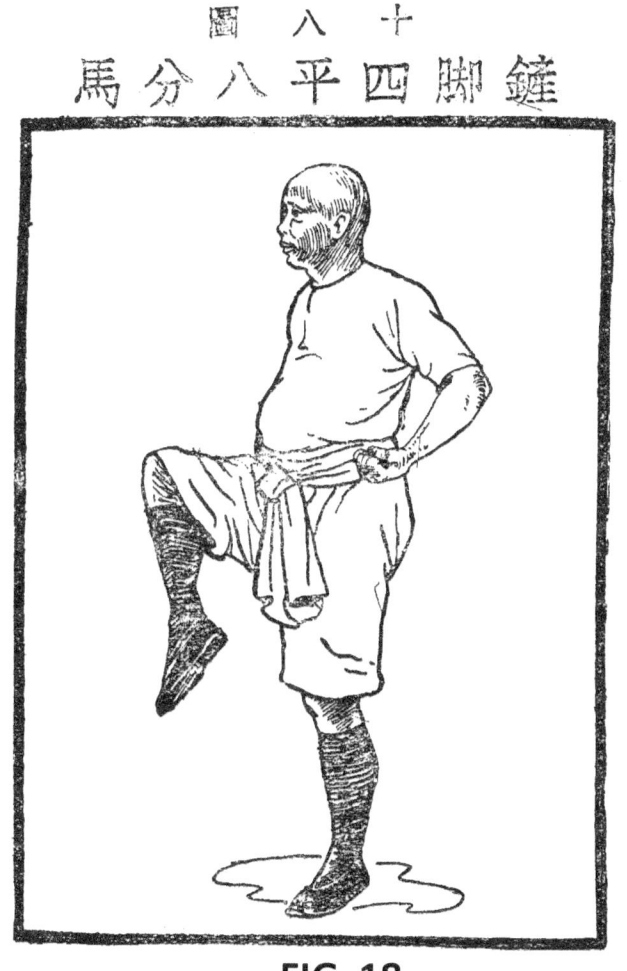

十八圖
馬分八平四腳鏟

一落四平八分馬倘敵人用中拳打來我即將腳一轉
子午馬用單膀手法破之

FIG. 18

十九 子午連轉單膀手

ZI WU LIAN ZHUAN DAN BO SHOU (Mandarin)
JI NG LIN JYUN DAAN BONG SAU (Cantonese)

19. Use One Arm Continuously in the Stance JI NG.

I use the inner part of my forearm and proceed from the movement BONG SAU[I] with one arm from outside to inside to the movement from inside to outside. I should "cut" the enemy's arm with my forearm from outside to inside and immediately "build a bridge" from inside to outside, i.e., a blow or blocking with the outer side of the forearm.

Commentaries: When you are in the position shown in **Fig. 19**, you block an enemy's blow at the middle level with a circular movement of your left forearm from inside to outside. Bring your right fist to the body, then make a turn round on your right foot and take the position shown in **Fig. 20**. Without stopping, block an enemy's blow on your head with your left arm moving upward from down (your forearm is in the horizontal plane at the level of your forehead, your palm is open and faces the front).

[I] *"Arm Like a Wing"* (膀手, Mandarin: ***BANG SHOU***, Cantonese: ***BONG SAU***), a forearm block, **[see index, p. 215]**.

十九圖

子午連轉單膀手

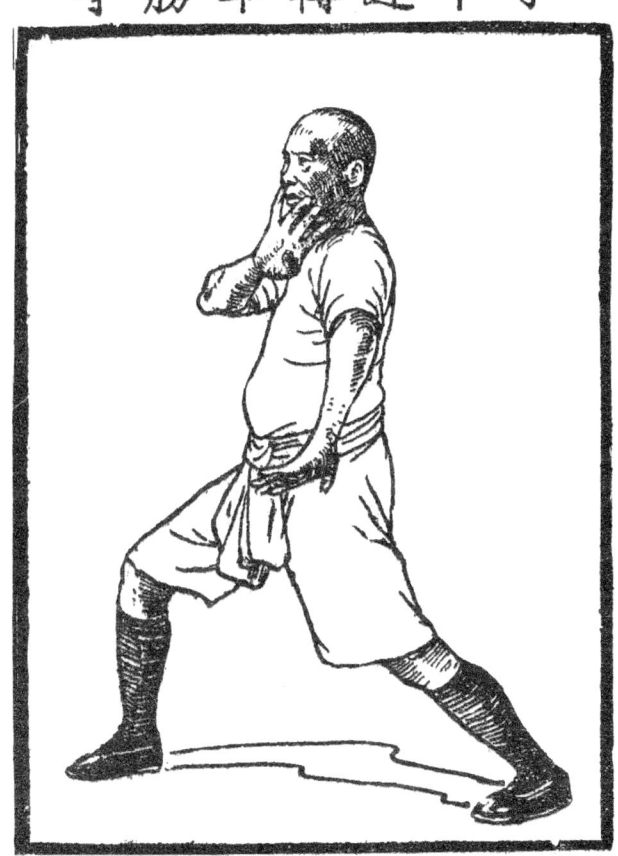

此法即內膀手法膀手有內外之分單膀即內膀割手
即外膀若與敵人搭橋橋來橋上過馬到馬發標

FIG. 19

二十　一挑擰馬千字落

YI TIAO NING MA QIAN ZI LUO (Mandarin)
JAT TIU NING MAA CIN JI LOK (Cantonese)

20. Throw a Thrust, Twist into the MAA Stance, the Falling Hand of 1000 Characters.

First, it is necessary to beat off the enemy's attack using the "Hand of 1000 Characters."[I] Then, to deliver a cutting blow, it means attacking with the "Hand of 1000 Characters." If the enemy retreats and answers with the "Paired Overhanging Fist"[II], striking on my arm and elbow from up to down, I "pull out" my fists and immediately use both "piercing hands" BIU CYUN SAU[III] to attack him.

Commentaries: In this case, you use your left arm. At first, with a waving downward movement from the top, you parry an enemy's attack on the middle level, then you pass on to the stance ***JI NG MAA*** (**Fig. 19**) and deliver a "cutting" blow with the side of your forearm and your palm from inside to outside. The palm is open and turned upward. It is ***"Hand of a Thousand Characters"*** that is used. The movements are fast

---

[I] *"The Hand of 1000 Characters"* (千字手, Mandarin: **QIAN ZI SHOU**, Cantonese: **CIN JI SAU**) - a wide range of blows and blocking with the arm (forearm), both from the inside out and the outside in, at different angles to the line of attack. The variations of this technique are shown in **Figs. 29, 35, 38, 42 [see index, p. 219]**. See also: *Lam Sai Wing, **"Tiger and Crane"***.

[II] *"Paired Overhanging Fist"* (雙掛拳, Mandarin: **SHUANG GUA QUAN**, Cantonese: **SEUNG GWA KYUN**) - simultaneous blows (or a block) with the backsides of both fists and (or) the outer sides of forearms delivered from up to down. The fists move from the forehead level forward and down to the chest level **[index, p. 222]**.

[III] *"Do a Mark with a Piercing Hand"* (標串手, Mandarin: **BIAO CHUAN SHOU**, Cantonese: **BIU CYUN SAU**) - a thrusting blow with the ends of fingers of an open palm **[index, p. 217]**.

and strong; it is necessary to use the force of the waist (to "twist" your body). When blocking a blow, slightly incline your body to the front and turn it to the right; when delivering a cutting blow to the outside, use your back muscles.

二 十 圖
一 挑 撐 馬 千 字 落

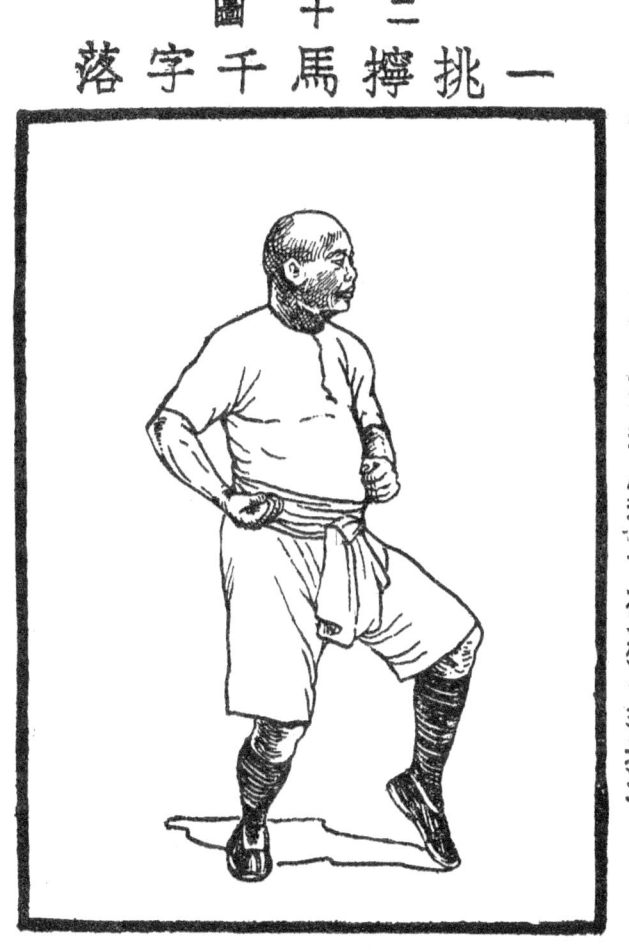

舉千字手一撤雙手一劃即攻千手抽拳歸後雙掛拳
是為千字手偏敵人托我胜我即用雙標串手招之

FIG. 20

廿一　抽手轉身割歸後

CHOU SHOU ZHUAN SHEN GE GUI HOU (Mandarin)
CAU SAU JYUN SAN GOT GWAI HAU (Cantonese)

21. Pull Back the Hand, Turn the Torso, Cut, and Come Back.

Pull back your hand and cut. If the enemy attacks from the side, instantly pull back your hand after the previous attack, turn on your left foot, and assume a "Scissor Stance"[I]. At the same time, with the hand passing near the head, "cut" the enemy's attack. Then, deliver a flank blow with your palm without interrupting the movement.

Commentaries: You turn about on your left foot clockwise and take the position shown in **Fig. 21**. Simultaneously, you parry an enemy's attack from the right with your left hand and forearm. Then, without stopping, you move forward to the position *JI NG MAA* ("Bow and Arrow") and deliver a blow with your palm on an enemy's side (**Fig. 22**).

[I] *"Scissor Stance"* (剪馬, Mandarin: *JIAN MA*, Cantonese: *ZIN MAA*) - this position is shown in **Fig. 21 [index, p. 224]**.

抽手割後之法若敵人由側打來我用手一抽招之由
後打來我將左脚敗回較剪馬將手過頭一割消之連
環一側掌打出

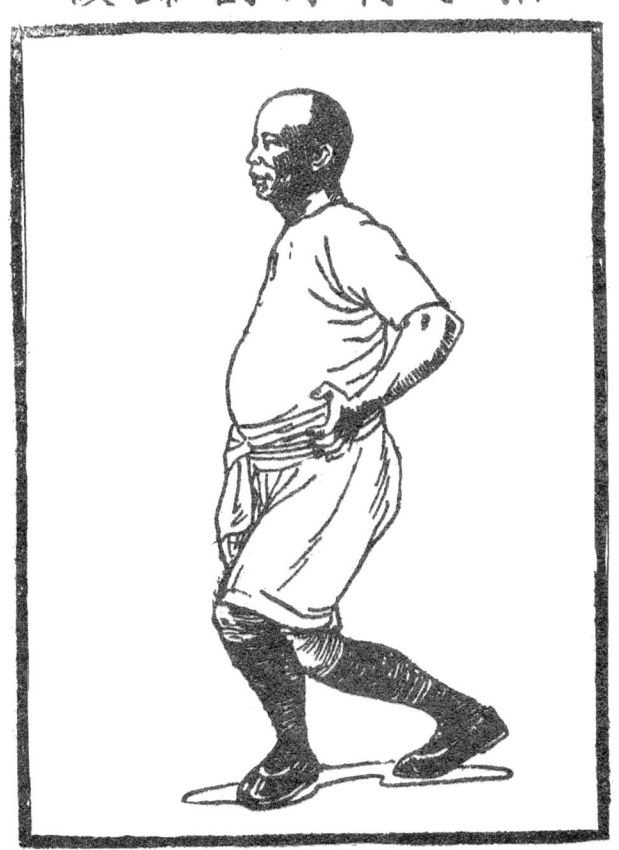

FIG. 21

廿二　上馬連變側掌打

SHANG MA LIAN BIAN QIE ZHANG DA (Mandarin)
SOENG MAA LIN BIN ZAK JEUNG DAA (Cantonese)

22. Riding a Horse, Smoothly Change Position and Deliver a Blow Aside with Your Palm.

If my blow with a palm aside is missed, the enemy can use a gap in my defense to attack me. I at once "tighten the bridle rein of the General's Horse", turn my torso and retreat to the stance SEI PING MAA[I]. At the same time, I bend my right arm and block the enemy's attack with my right forearm. Then, I use my palm again and deliver a "piercing blow" BIAO CHUAN SHOU[II].

Commentaries: If the enemy parries your blow and counterattacks with a blow to your head, it is necessary to pass on to the "Horse Stance" and, in this way, shift your body from the line of the attack. At the same time, with your left forearm, you deflect the enemy's blow aside (**Fig. 23**). Then, without stopping the movement, deliver **BIAO CHUAN SHOU** on the enemy's face or throat with your left arm. The position in **Fig. 23** can be regarded as a blow with your elbow to the enemy standing behind. It is an example of the multi-purpose use of fighting Kung Fu techniques.

[I] *"Horse Riding Stance"* (四平馬, Mandarin: *SEI PING MA*, Cantonese: *SEI PING MAA*) – literally: *"Four Levels Horse Stance"*, also known as the *"Horse Stance"* (馬步, *MA BU*) (Fig. 10), [see index, p. 220].

[II] *"Do a Mark with a Piercing Hand"* (標串手, Mandarin: *BIAO CHUAN SHOU*, Cantonese: *BIU CYUN SAU*) - a thrusting blow with the ends of fingers of an open palm [index, p. 217].

廿二圖

上馬連變側掌打

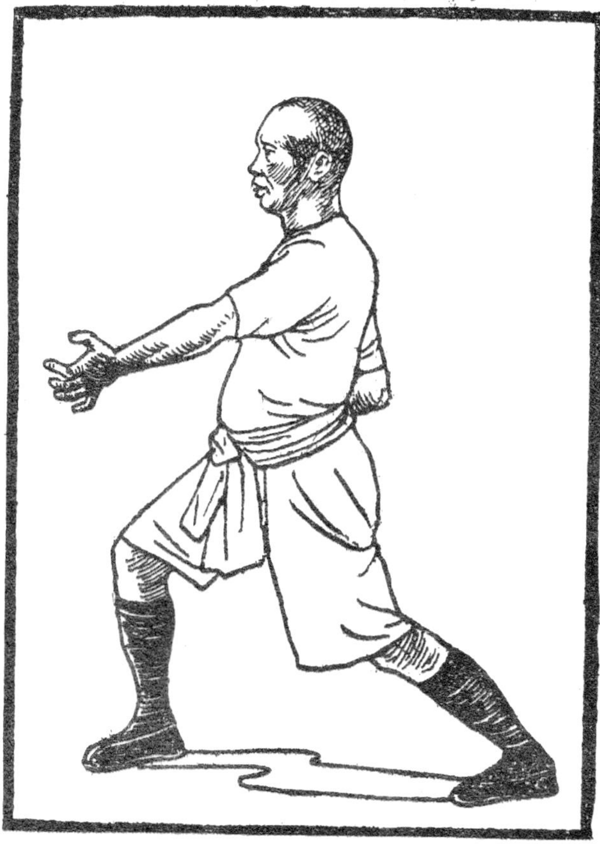

逢出側掌腰夾必空敵人由空而入我即將馬一拉轉回四平連變一頂膊再用標串手法攻之

FIG. 22

廿三　四平靜頂標串出

SEI PING ZHENG DING BIAO CHUAN CHU (Mandarin)
SEI PING ZAANG DENG BIU CYUN CHEUT (Cantonese)

23. SEI PING Stance, Push with the Tip of the Elbow, Piercing Blow.

If the enemy beats off my blow and continues attacking me with his elbow, I immediately retreat to the stance SEI PING MAA and "follow" his attack with my elbow. In other words, I "remove one elbow with another." This is an "elbow against elbow" technique.

Commentaries: Here, the universality of techniques is stressed, one of the most important aspects of fighting Kung Fu. In other words, whichever method the enemy uses to deliver a blow (in this case, with a fist or an elbow), passing on to the **SEI PING MAA** ("Horse Stance") and parrying with an elbow allows you to avoid his blow and to counterattack immediately.

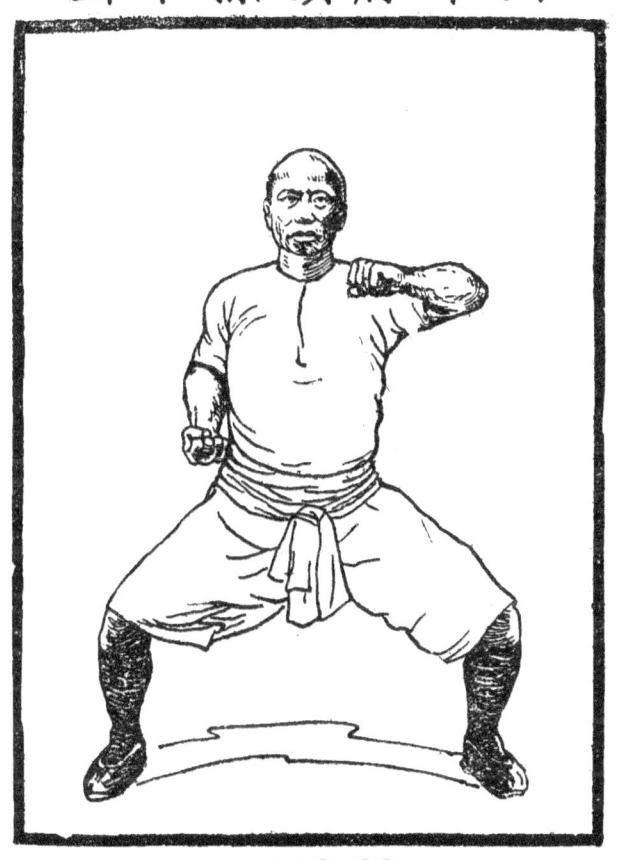

廿 三 圖

四平睜頂標串出

頂睜之法他用睜招我連用睜頂來我即以扭馬轉身
一磋睜招之此乃以睜消睜之法也

FIG. 23

廿四　割手四平掌打正

GE SHOU SEI PING ZHANG DA ZHENG (Mandarin)
GOT SAU SEI PING ZEUNG DAA ZING (Cantonese)

24. Cut with a Hand, SEI PING Stance, Straight Blow with a Palm.

If the enemy attacks me from a side or from behind, I immediately turn to the stance SEI PING MAA and, at the same time, use GOT SAU[I] to "cut" his attacking arm with my palm. Then, without interrupting the movement, I deliver a blow with my palm to the center of his breast. If the enemy tries to catch my wrist, I sharply pull my hand and free myself from a clench.

Commentaries: After striking with your fingertips (***BIAO CHUAN SHOU***) in the stance ***JI NG MAA*** (or "Bow and Arrow", this phase is not shown in the figures but is present in the text), turn to the left and take the ***SEI PING MAA*** ("Horse Stance"). Your left palm moves to the waist, then you deliver a blow with "tiger's claws" (**Fig. 24**). The repulse of the enemy's attack and your subsequent blow are done with your left hand. You must act swiftly and forestall the enemy. However, force should not be sacrificed to speed. If your blow is not strong enough, the enemy will go on attacking, and you will find yourself in a dangerous position. Force and speed are two essential requirements in fighting Kung Fu.

[I] *"Cutting Hand"* (割手, Mandarin: ***GE SHOU***, Cantonese: ***GOT SAU***) - cutting block with the edge of the palm, the movement is directed from top to bottom [index, p. 216].

廿 四 圖
割手四平掌打正

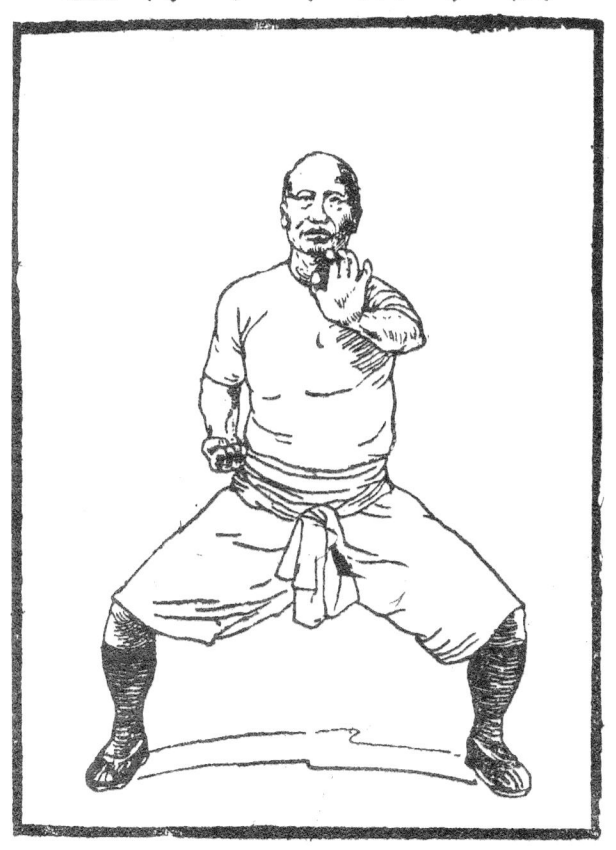

此勢倘敵人由腰部攻入我卽立正四平馬一割連環
一掌打正他心胸他若搶我手腕我卽將拳一抽一分
救之

FIG. 24

25. Clench the Fist, Pull Out the Hand, Turn and Split.

"The Gold-Splitting Fist"[I] is used if the enemy attacks you with his fist. Immediately use "The Gold-Splitting Fist" and eliminate his attack without fail. FEN JIN means "to split gold", in other words, to obtain "The Five Elements" (WU XING)[II]: Metal, Wood, Water, Fire, and Earth. Which particular punch corresponds to each element of WU XING? WU XING includes JIN QUAN ("Metal (Gold) Fist"), MU QUAN ("Wooden Fist"), SHUI LANG QUAN ("Water Stream Fist"), HUO JIAN QUAN ("Fire Fist like a Rocket"), TU PAO QUAN ("Fist Flinging from the Earth").

Commentaries: If the enemy grips your hand at the moment of your striking on his breast (**Fig. 4**), it is necessary to clench the gripped hand into a fist and "tear" it out of the enemy's grip with a sharp jerk to the center of your breast, thus you free yourself from the grip. Then, without interrupting the movement, you deliver the blow ***GWA***[III] on the head or the breast of the enemy with the same arm. Then you pull the fist

---

[I] **"The Gold-Splitting Fist"** (分金拳, Mandarin: **FEN JIN QUAN**, Cantonese: **FAN GAM KYUN**) - Pull your fist toward the center of your chest, then lower your fist out to the side to waist level. In the final position, the back of the fist faces the earth, the elbow is slightly bent and placed near the side, and the forearm is in a horizontal plane **[index, p. 218]**.

[II] **Five Elements** (五行, Mandarin: **WU XING**, Cantonese: **NG HANG**) - the five primordial (basic) elements, a fundamental concept in Chinese philosophy and cosmology: **Wood, Fire, Earth, Metal**, and **Water [index, p. 218]**.

[III] **"Overhanging Fist"** (掛拳, Mandarin: **GUA QUAN**, Cantonese: **GWA KYUN**) - blow (or a block) with the back side of the fist and (or) the outer side of the forearm delivered from up to down. The fist moves from the shoulder level to the waist, making a semi-circle in the vertical plane **[index, p. 222]**.

to your chest and pass to the **"Gold-Splitting Fist"**, i.e., lower the fist through the side to the waist level. In the final position, the back side of the fist faces the earth, the elbow is slightly bent and placed near your waist, and the forearm is located in the horizontal plane. All the movements are done in the stance **SEI PING MAA** ("Horse"). The execution of the technique **"The Gold-Splitting Fist"** is very close to the method **"Dividing the Gold Bridge"** (**Fig. 16**). The only difference is that the fist, in this case, moves not in the horizontal but in the vertical plane.

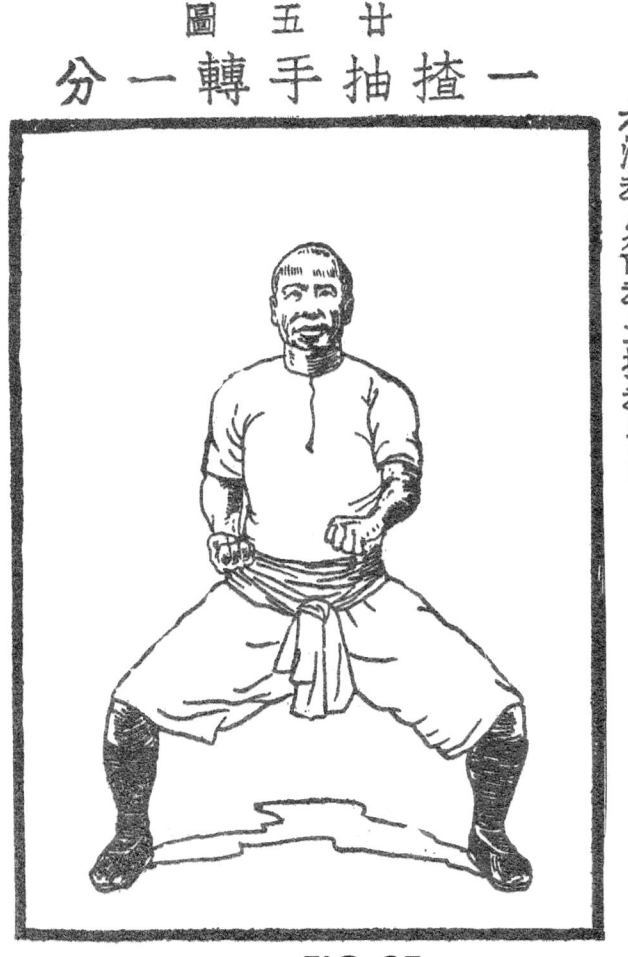

圖 五 廿
分 一 轉 手 抽 揸 一

分金拳勢倘敵人一拳打來我即用分金拳連消帶打
招之分金乃五行拳法之一何謂五行分金拳夾木拳
水浪拳火箭拳土拋拳是也

FIG. 25

廿六　出右吊左拉歸後

CHU YOU DIAO ZUO LA GUI HOU (Mandarin)
CHEUT JAU DIU JO LAAI GWAI HAU (Cantonese)

26. Go Out to the Right, Hang on the Left, Pull Up and Come Back.

I step with my right foot, my left foot pulls back and returns, and my torso turns to the left. I raise my left foot. If the enemy kicks me, I immediately stop his attack with my foot, so the foot uses force to another foot.

Commentaries: From this position, the techniques shown in **Figs. 17 - 25** are performed in the opposite direction: turn left (left-side stance), left kick, etc. (**Figs. 26 - 34**).

See commentaries to **Fig. 17**.

廿六圖
出右吊左拉歸後

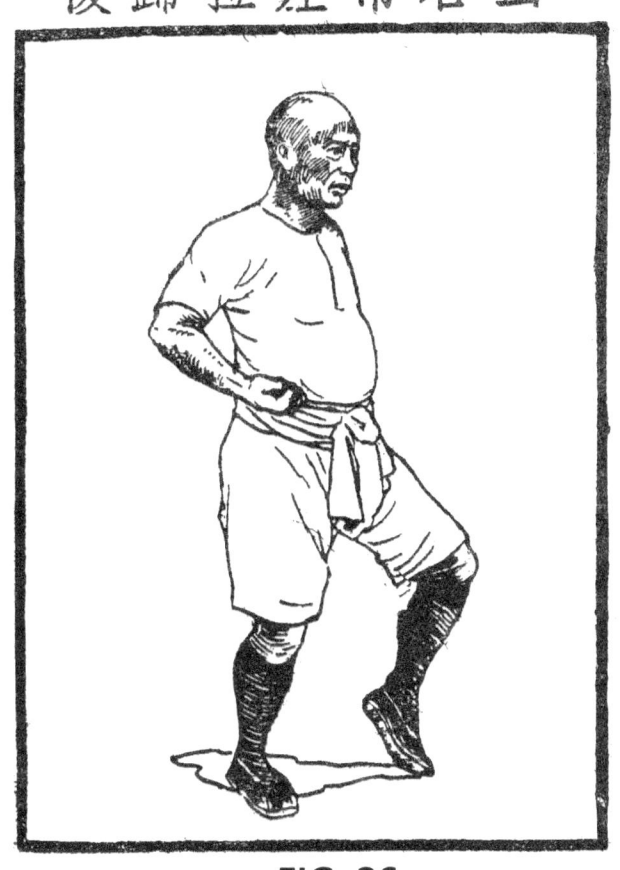

右脚一踏出將左脚拉歸後身向左將脚一起偷他人
用脚打來我即用脚消之即以脚消脚之法

FIG. 26

廿七 鏟脚四平馬八分

CHAN JIAO SEI PING MA BA FEN (Mandarin)
CHAN GEUK SEI PING MAA BAAT FAN (Cantonese)

27. A Foot Like a Spade, Lower to the Stance SEI PING BA FEN MA.

I am in the stance SEI PING BAAT FAN MAA[I]. The enemy punches me on the middle level from the side. I immediately turn and take the stance JI NG MAA[II], repel the attack with one arm, "pull out" my hand, turn into MAA DIU GEUK[III], deliver a blow, and pull my hand back.

Commentaries: See commentaries to **Fig. 18**.

[I] *"Horse Riding Stance"* (四平馬, Mandarin: *SEI PING MA*, Cantonese: *SEI PING MAA*) – literally: *"Four Levels Horse Stance"*, also known as the *"Horse Stance"* (馬步, *MA BU*) **(Fig. 10)**, **[index, p. 220]**.

[II] *JI NG MAA*, 子午馬 **(Figs. 28, 29)**, or *"Bow and Arrow Stance"* **[see index, p. 220]**.

[III] *"Hanging Foot Stance"* (馬吊腳, Mandarin: *MA DIAO JIAO*, Cantonese: *MAA DIU GEUK*) - known in modern *WUSHU* as the *"Cat's Stance"* **(Fig. 26)**. The term *"MAA"* is used in the meaning "a stance" here **[index p. 219]**.

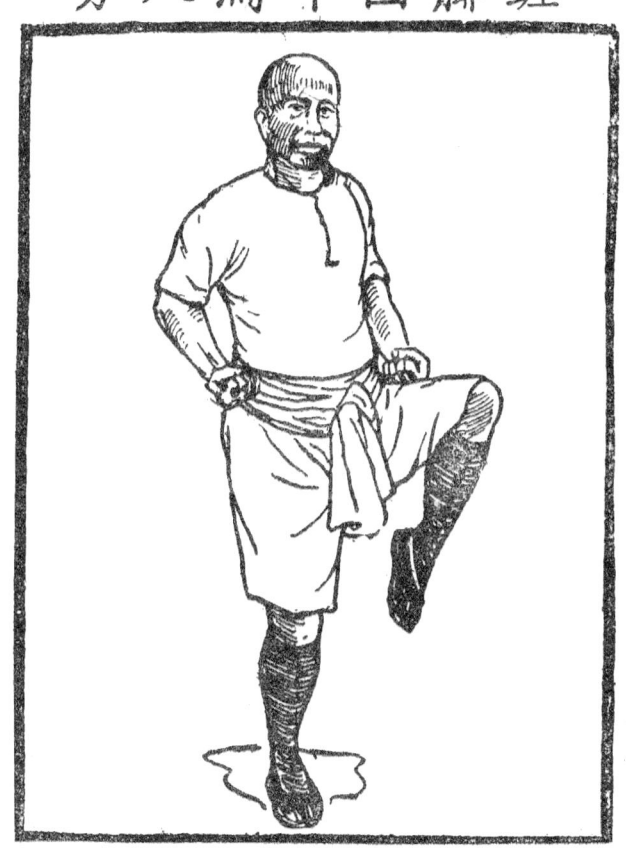

廿七圖

鏟腳四平馬八分

四平八分馬敵人一拳由中部打來我即轉子午馬用單膀手招之抽手擰馬吊腳一撳又一抽

FIG. 27

廿八　子午一轉右膀手

ZI WU YI ZHUAN YOU BANG SHOU (Mandarin)
JI NG JAT JYUN JAU BONG SAU (Cantonese)

28. Turn to the JI NG Stance, Blocking with the Right Forearm.

If the enemy punches me to the middle part, I immediately block it with the "Arm Like a Wing"[I] technique. If he punches me again, I deliver a sharp cutting blow from up to down obliquely, "hang up" my left foot[II], and go on with the method "Hand of 1000 Characters"[III].

Commentaries: See commentaries to **Fig. 19.**

[I] ***"Arm Like a Wing"*** (膀手, Mandarin: ***BANG SHOU***, Cantonese: ***BONG SAU***), a forearm block, **[see index, p. 215]**.

[II] This refers to the ***"Hanging Foot Stance"*** (馬吊腳, Mandarin: ***MA DIAO JIAO***, Cantonese: ***MAA DIU GEUK***), see **Fig. 26**.

[III] ***"The Hand of 1000 Characters"*** (千字手, Mandarin: ***QIAN ZI SHOU***, Cantonese: ***CIN JI SAU***) - a wide range of blows and blocking with the arm (forearm), both from the inside out and the outside in, at different angles to the line of attack. The variations of this technique are shown in **Figs. 29, 35, 38, 42 [see index, p. 219]**. See also: *Lam Sai Wing*, ***"Tiger and Crane"***.

子午一轉右膀手

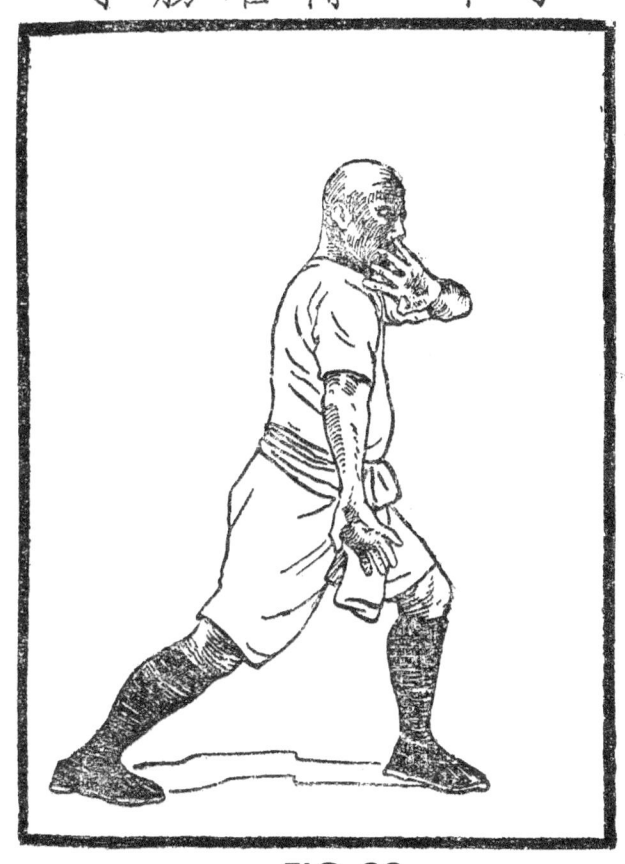

此勢如敵人一中拳打來我即用膀手招之再用拳打
來我用抽劈手吊左脚連用千字手法

FIG. 28

廿九 一挑擰馬右千字

YI TIAO NING MA YOU QIAN ZI (Mandarin)
JAT TIU NING MAA JAU CIN JI (Cantonese)

29. Throw a Thrust, Twist into the MAA Stance, the Right Hand of 1000 Characters.

If the enemy attacks me from behind, I turn around, pull my right foot back, raise my right hand above my head, and immediately block the blow from the other side - the palm cuts from above, moving to the left hip. I straighten my trunk and stop the opponent's piercing strike BIU CYUN[I], deflecting his arm to the right.

Commentaries: See commentaries to **Fig. 20**.

_____

[I] ***"Do a Mark with a Piercing Hand"*** (標串掌, Mandarin: ***BIAO CHUAN ZHANG***, Cantonese: ***BIU CYUN JEUNG***) - a thrust blow with the ends of fingers of an open palm **[see index, p. 217].**

廿九圖

一挑擰馬右千字

如敵人由後打來我即將右脚歸後左手過頭劏下一側掌將左脚搕正一頂脖標串掌一劏打正

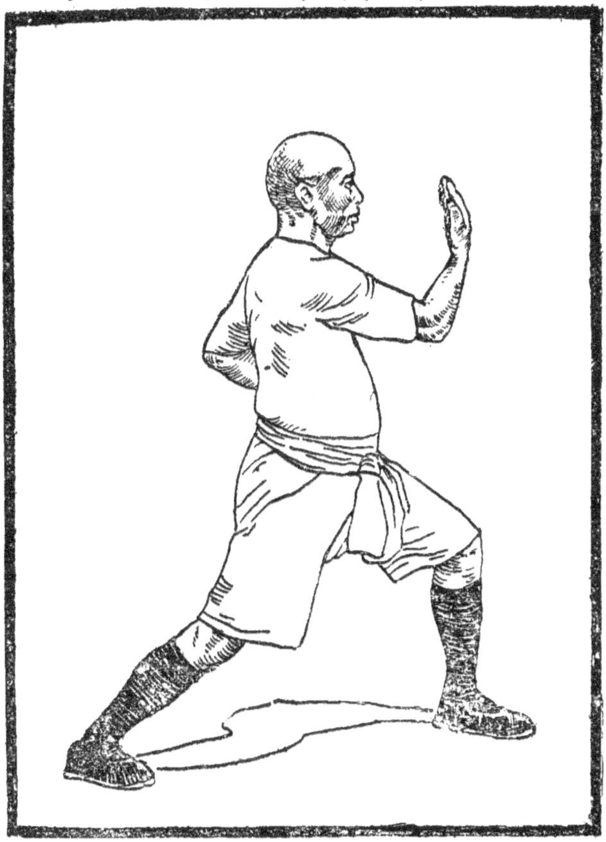

FIG. 29

三十　抽手轉身割歸後

CHOU SHOU ZHUAN SHEN GE GUI HOU (Mandarin)
CAU SAU JYUN SAN GOT GWAI HAU (Cantonese)

30. Pull Out a Hand, Turn the Torso, "Cut," and Come Back.

If the enemy attacks me with a punch, I use the method "To turn the torso and to cut with a hand." I immediately "cut" with a hand[I], twist, and simultaneously step back, followed by a blow to the enemy's side. I strike with my elbow and "Do a Mark with a Piercing Hand"[II] - one after the other.

Commentaries: See commentaries to **Fig. 21**.

[I] *"Cutting Hand"* (割手, Mandarin: **GE SHOU**, Cantonese: **GOT SAU**) - Cutting block with the edge of the palm, the movement is directed from top to bottom **[see index, p. 216]**.

[II] *"Do a Mark with a Piercing Hand"* (標串手, Mandarin: **BIAO CHUAN SHOU**, Cantonese: **BIU CYUN SAU**) - **[see index, p. 217]**.

三十圖

抽手轉身割歸後

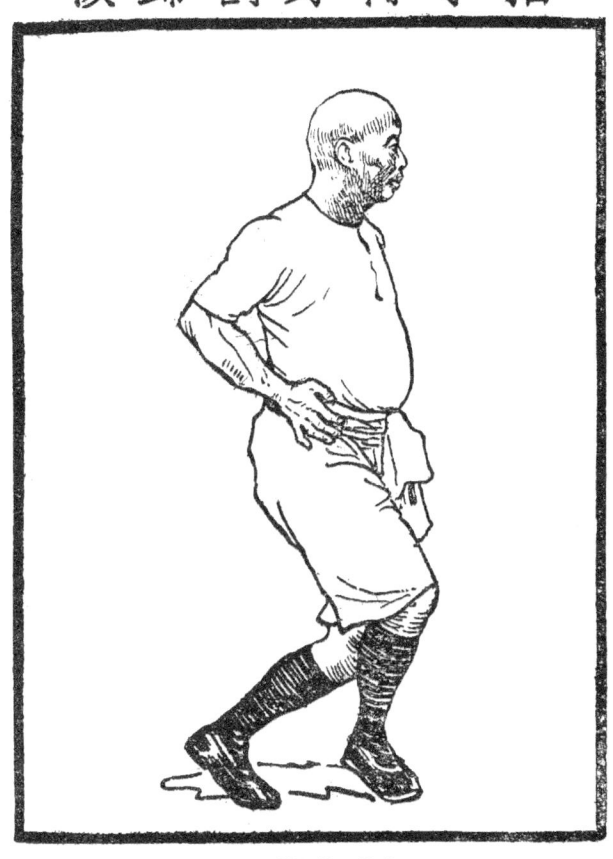

FIG. 30

轉身割手之法如敵人一拳打來我即將手一割攬後
連環側掌打出即用頂膞標串手法

卅一　上馬連出一側掌

SHANG MA LIAN CHU YI QE ZHANG (Mandarin)
SOENG MAA LIN CHEUT JAT ZAK JEUNG (Cantonese)

31. To Mount the Horse, to Deliver a Blow to the Side with the Palm.

The method of "Side Palm"[I] means an attack directed to the enemy's side, namely to his waist region. If the enemy attacks me from behind, I "submerge" into the firm position SEI PING MA and execute the elbow-tip blow technique followed by techniques "Do a Mark with a Piercing Hand" (BIU CYUN SAU) [II], "Cutting Hand" (GOT SAU)[III], and "Make a Grip" (ZAA)[IV].

Commentaries: See commentaries to **Fig. 22**.

[I] *"Side Palm"* (側掌, Mandarin: **QE ZHANG**, Cantonese: **JAK JEUNG**) - a blow with the heel of an open palm, fingers turned outward, **Fig. 31**, **[index, p. 224]**.

[II] *"Do a Mark with a Piercing Hand"* (標串掌, Mandarin: **BIAO CHUAN ZHANG**, Cantonese: **BIU CYUN JEUNG**), **(Fig. 32)**, **[see index, p. 217]**.

[III] See **Fig. 33**.

[IV] See **Fig. 34**.

上馬連出一側掌

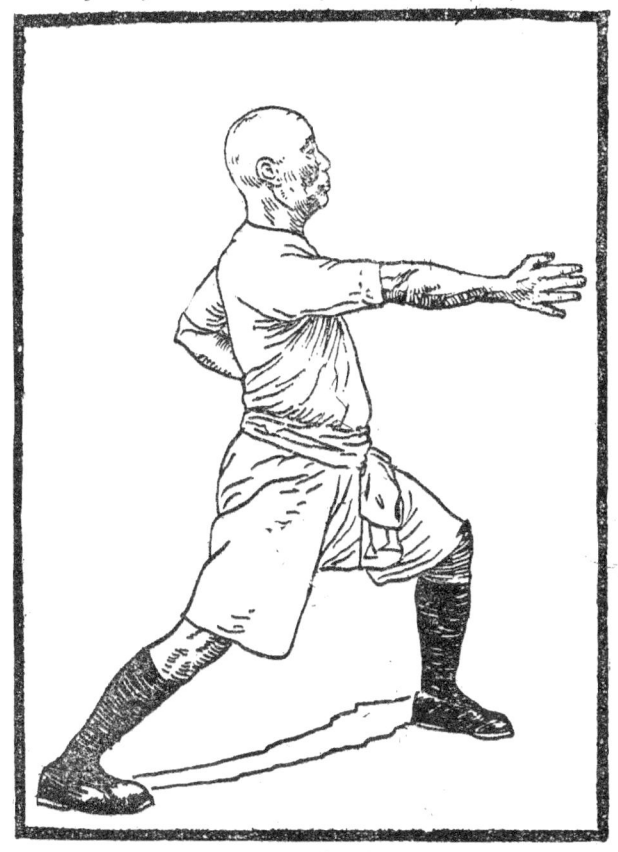

側掌之法打敵人之腰部倘由後打來我落正四平馬一頂靜標串一割一揸分

FIG. 31

卅二　四平静頂標串手

SEI PING ZHENG DING BIAO CHUAN SHOU (Mandarin)
SEI PING ZAANG DENG BIU CYUN SAU (Cantonese)

32. SEI PING Stance, Push with the Tip of the Elbow, Piercing Hand.

A blow with the elbow tip in a stable position SEI PING MAA smoothly transforms into a piercing finger strike BIU CYUN[I]. If the enemy attacks me from the side, I immediately turn the torso into a firm position and "cut" (GOT) his blow, then deliver a strike with my palm, continue the movement, and make a grip (ZAA).

Commentaries: Here, the author lists **BIU CYUN** and the following techniques (see **Figs. 32, 33, 34**). See commentaries to **Fig. 23**.

[I] *"Do a Mark with a Piercing Hand"* (標串掌, Mandarin: **BIAO CHUAN ZHANG**, Cantonese: **BIU CYUN JEUNG**) - a thrust blow with the ends of fingers of an open palm **(Fig. 32), [index, p. 217]**.

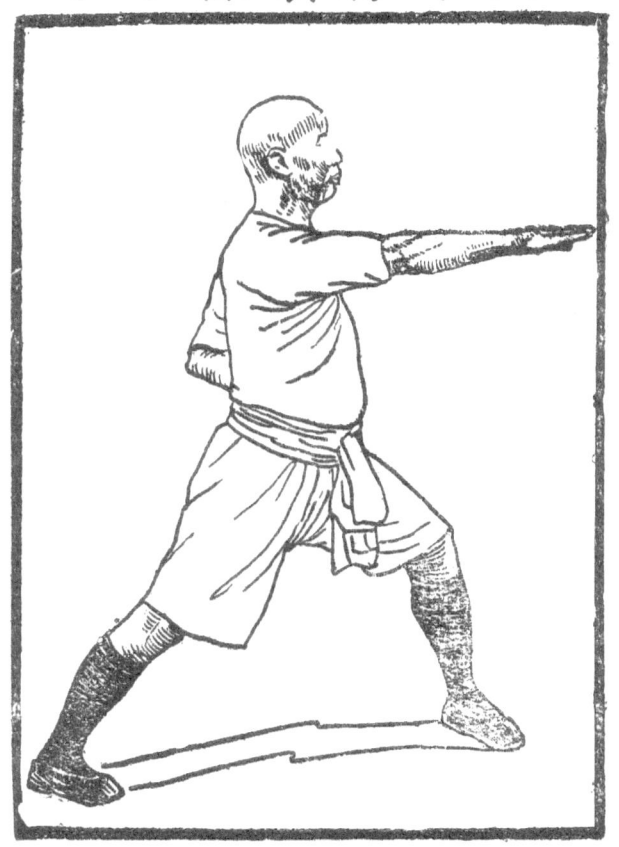

四平睜頂標串手　卅二圖

四平頂睜連環標串如敵人由腰部打來我即將身轉正一割一掌打出連轉一揸一分之法

FIG. 32

卅三　割手四平掌打正

GE SHOU SEI PING ZHANG DA ZHENG (Mandarin)
GOT SAU SEI PING JEUNG DAA ZING (Cantonese)

33. Cut with a Hand, SEI PING Stance, Straight Blow with a Palm.

The technique "Cutting Hand"[I] is used if the enemy punches me. I immediately lower myself into a firm position SEI PING MAA and deliver a blow with my palm[II]. If he uses the "Crossing Palm"[III] and deviates my blow with a push to my elbow, I attack his head (with another arm). If he caught my arm, I would pull my arm to myself[IV] to upset his equilibrium. In other words, "mount the horse and rein it".

Commentaries: See commentaries to **Fig. 24**.

[I] *"Cutting Hand"* (割手, Mandarin: *GE SHOU*, Cantonese: *GOT SAU*) - Cutting block with the edge of the palm, the movement is directed from top to bottom **[index, p. 216]**. See **Fig. 33**.

[II] See **Fig. 24** (in this case, the blow is delivered with the right palm).

[III] *"Crossing Palm"* (橫掌, Mandarin: *HENG ZHANG*, Cantonese: *WAANG JEUNG*) - a horizontal open palm block that deflects the strike to the side **[index, p. 216]**.

[IV] See **Fig. 34**.

卅三圖

割手四平掌打正

割手四平之法敵人一拳打來我即立正四平一掌打出他用橫掌伏我膊由頭部攻我我即用掌扱他膊上馬迫他

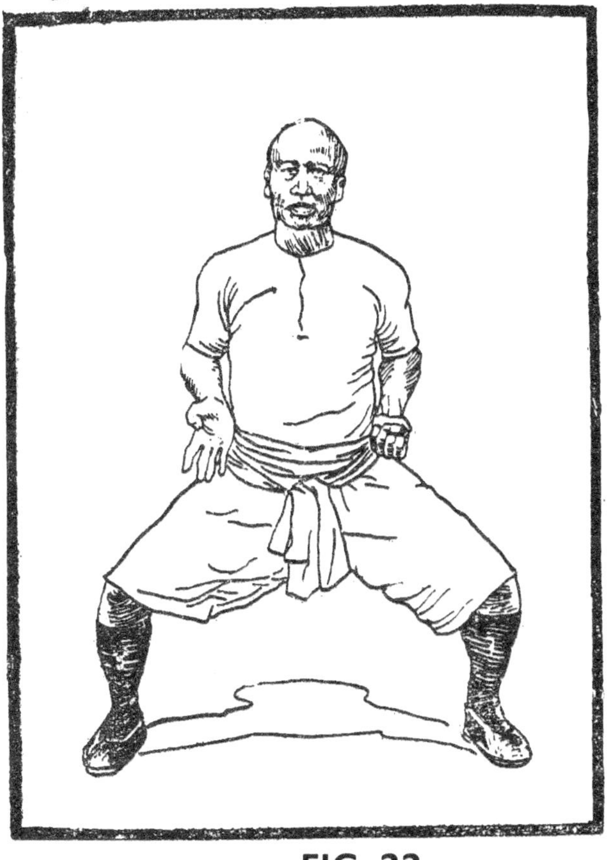

FIG. 33

卅四 一揸一抽轉一分

YI ZHA YI CHOU ZHUAN YI FEN (Mandarin)
JAT ZAA JAT CAU JYUN JAT FAN (Cantonese)

34. Clench the Fist, Grip and Pull Out, Turn and Split.

The enemy grabs my arm and pulls it towards himself. I pull inside (i.e., to myself), and then "spread" with my hands. This technique is called FAN GAM KYUN - "The Gold-Splitting Fist"[I], followed immediately by the GWA KYUN - "Overhanging Fist"[II]. If the enemy delivers a blow to my heart or my side with his fist, I "mount the horse" without delay, use the "Overhanging Fist," and stop his attack.

Commentaries: See commentaries to **Fig. 25**.

[I] *"The Gold-Splitting Fist"* (分金拳, Mandarin: **FEN JIN QUAN**, Cantonese: **FAN GAM KYUN**) - Pull your fist toward the center of your chest, then lower your fist out to the side to waist level. In the final position, the back of the fist faces the earth, the elbow is slightly bent and placed near the side, and the forearm is in a horizontal plane **[index, p. 218]**.

[II] *"Overhanging Fist"* (掛拳, Mandarin: **GUA QUAN**, Cantonese: **GWA KYUN**) - blow (or a block) with the back side of the fist and (or) the outer side of the forearm delivered from up to down. The fist moves from the shoulder level to the waist, making a semi-circle in the vertical plane **[index, p. 222]**.

一揸一抽轉一分

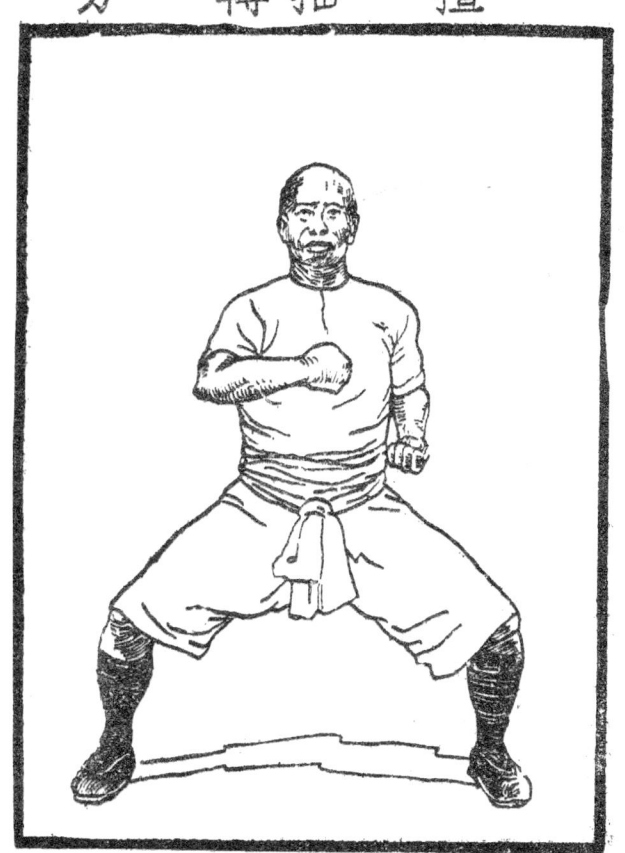

一揸之法即外膀一抽之法即內膀一分之法即金
拳法此法即掛拳也如敵人用拳打我心脅我即連環
上馬用掛拳消之

FIG. 34

卅五　出左踏右吊脚馬

CHU ZUO TA YOU DIAO JIAO MA (Mandarin)
CHEUT JO DAAP JAU DIU GEUK MAA (Cantonese)

35. Go Out to the Left, Hang the Foot on the Right, Take a Stance.

Step to the left, hang the foot on the right, then take the stance JI NG BAAT FAN MAA[I]. I should use the technique "Look at Yourself in a Hand Mirror"[II] to protect myself from a fist blow directed at me. Then, I immediately use "claws" and scratch the enemy's face three times in succession.

Commentaries: After the execution of the method **"Look at Yourself in a Hand Mirror"** (**Fig. 35**) with your right arm, immediately pass to the technique **"The Kitten Washes Its Muzzle"** (**Fig. 36**). The hands transform into **"Tiger's claws"**, the right arm delivers a "scratching" blow on the enemy's face, and the left arm protects the heart and the middle part of the body against a possible counterattack. At the moment when "claws" contact the enemy's face, the fingertips bend more inward towards the center of the palm, as if the fingers were catching and tearing the soft tissues. This position of the hands is shown in **Fig. 36**.

[I] *JI NG BAAT FAN MAA* (子午八分馬, Mandarin: *ZI WU BA FEN MA*, Cantonese: *JI NG BAAT FAN MAA*) – literally: *"Four Levels JI NG Stance"* - lower *"Bow and Arrow"* stance, i.e., the feet are widespread, the center of gravity is situated low (**Fig. 36**), **[index, p. 220]**.

[II] *"Look at Yourself in a Hand Mirror"* (照鏡手法, Mandarin: *ZHAO JING SHOU FA*, Cantonese: *ZIU GENG SAU FAAT*) – a blocking movement with the side of the forearm from the inside to outside, in the final phase the palm is open and placed in front of your face (**Fig. 35**), **[index, p. 221]**.

馬脚吊右踏左出

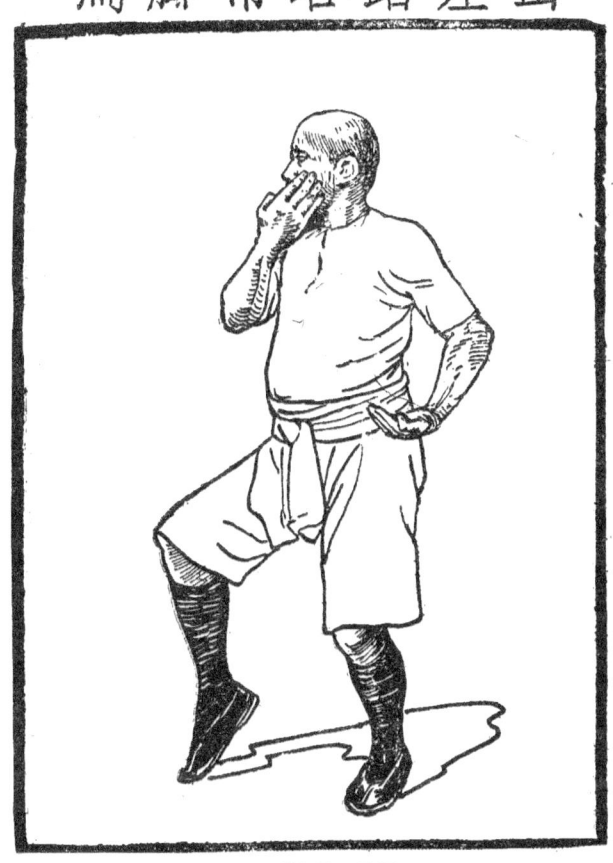

出左吊右子午八分馬照鏡手法防敵人用一拳打來
我即用爪連環三爪爪他面門

FIG. 35

卅六　照鏡手法爪三勻

ZHAO JING SHOU FA ZHAO SAN YUN (Mandarin)
ZIU GENG SAU FAAT ZAAU SAAM WAN (Cantonese)

36. Look at Yourself in a Hand Mirror, Three Claws in a Row.

In this position, if the enemy attacks me with his fist, I will use the technique "The Kitten Washes Its Muzzle."[I] I should hit three times and pull three times. Then I pull the enemy towards me. This method is called "To Take the Horse by the Bridle and Bring It Back to the Stall."[II]

Commentaries: You linger for a short while in the posture shown in **Fig. 36**, then shift the weight of your body on your back leg and take the **"Hanging Foot Stance"** (or *"The Cat's Stance,"* **Fig. 35**). The hands in the position **"Tiger's claws"** are drawn to the left side of the waist. Without stopping the movement, your right leg makes a step forward. You take the stance **JI NG MAA** (or *"The Bow and the Arrow"*) and carry out the method **"The Kitten Washes Its Muzzle"** (**Fig. 36**). If the enemy attacks you with his fist at your head or your breast, deflect his blow aside with your right forearm and, at the same time, attack his face with the "claws." One of the peculiarities of the old fighting Kung Fu was that there was no artificial division into blows and blocks. Any technique could be both

---

[I] *"The Kitten Washes Its Muzzle"* (貓兒洗面, Mandarin: *MAO ER XI MIAN*, Cantonese: *MAAU JI SAI MIN*) – Scratching motion with both hands from top to bottom and towards you. One arm is slightly extended forward, and the second hand is located at the elbow of the first. Attacking the opponent's face with the "tiger's claws" while simultaneously blocking his counter-punch (**Fig. 36**), **[index, p. 221]**.

[II] *"To Take the Horse by the Bridle and Bring It Back to the Stall"* (帶馬歸槽拉, Mandarin: *DAI MA GUI CAO LA*, Cantonese: *DAAI MAA GWAI COU LAAI*) – i.e., to catch the enemy's clothes and to pull him towards yourself, at the same time to move the body back and to shift the center of gravity to the back supporting leg (**Fig. 37**), **[index, p. 226]**.

strike and block at the same time. In a moment, one movement transformed into another, which left no chance for an inexperienced enemy.

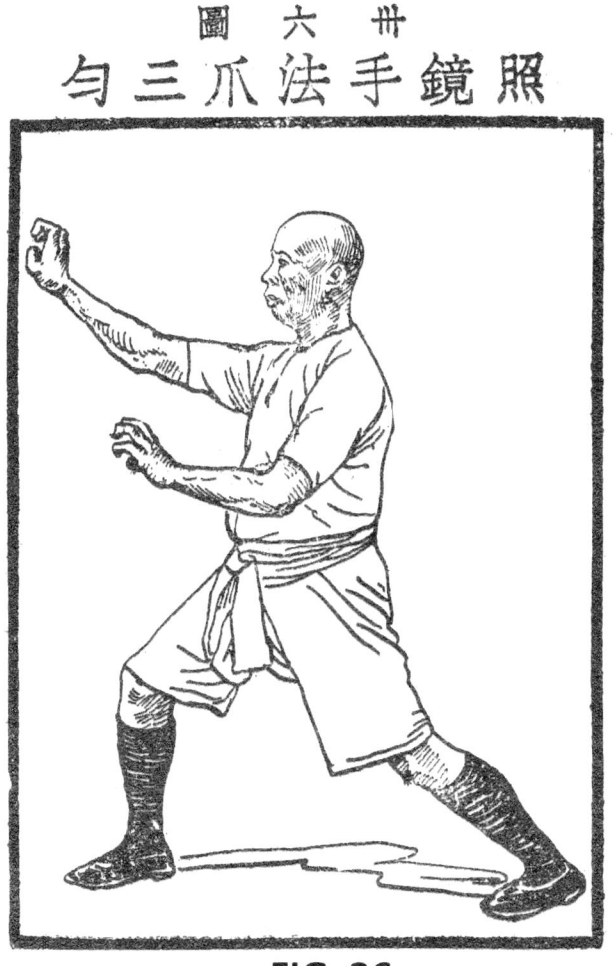

照鏡手法爪三勻

卅六圖

此勢若敵人用拳打來我即用貓兒洗面之法三打三招運用帶馬歸槽拉敵人歸後

FIG. 36

DAI MA GUI CAO LA ZHUAN HOU (Mandarin)
DAAI MAA GWAI COU LAAI JYUN HAU (Cantonese)

37. To Take the Horse by the Bridle and Bring It Back to the Stall, Pull and Turn Back.

When using the technique "To Take the Horse by the Bridle and Bring It Back to the Stall," it is necessary to straighten and strain the back leg when turning back. I turn around into a stance JI NG MAA and pull the enemy towards me like a tortoise raking up sand.

Commentaries: After you have executed the technique ***"The Kitten Washes Its Muzzle"*** three times, take the ***"Hanging Foot Stance"*** (or *"The Cat's Stance"*) and lower your "claws" to the left knee. Here, another variant of this technique is that you beat off the attacking arm of the enemy and immediately grab it with your "claws" in the region of the wrist and the elbow bent. Then you pull your enemy to yourself and down and retreat to the ***"Hanging Foot Stance."*** Then, your right leg makes a step forward to take the stance ***JI NG MAA*** (or *"The Bow and the Arrow"*), and you deliver a blow to the enemy's head with both your arms (the hands are left in the position "claws"). Then you clench your hands into fists, pull them with strain to the breast, and turn 180 degrees. This position is shown in **Fig. 37:** after catching the enemy's clothes, you pull him to yourself to upset his balance. It is the final position of the technique ***"To Take the Horse by the Bridle and Bring It Back to the Stall."***

卅七圖

帶馬歸槽拉轉後

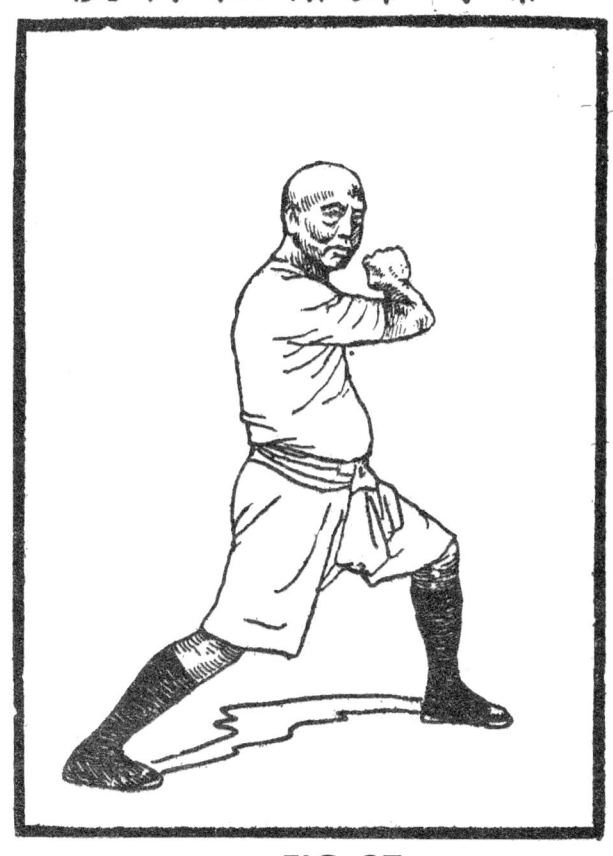

帶馬歸槽之法須要拉後脚轉子午馬將敵人一拉如烏龜扒沙一般

FIG. 37

卅八　貓兒洗面又三勻

MAO ER XI MIAN YOU SAN YUN (Mandarin)
MAAU JI SAI MIN JAU SAAM WAN (Cantonese)

38. The Kitten Washes Its Muzzle Again, Three Times in a Row.

I should meet the enemy with the technique "Look at Yourself in a Hand Mirror,"[I] take the stance JI NG MAA at once, and go on with the method "The Kitten Washes Its Muzzle"[II] with the use of the "claws". It is necessary that the "claws" (of the back arm) and the elbow (of the front arm) should be at the breast level and the "claws" (of the front arm) against the nose. Then, I continue with the technique "To Take the Horse by the Bridle and Bring It Back to the Stall."

Commentaries: From the position shown in **Fig. 37,** you shift the body weight to your back leg and take the **"Hanging Foot Stance"** (or *"The Cat's Stance"*). At the same time, you carry out the technique ***Look at Yourself in a Hand Mirror"*** with your left arm (**Fig. 38**). Then you execute the method ***"The Kitten Washes Its Muzzle"*** three times (now in the left side stance).

_____

[I] *"Look at Yourself in a Hand Mirror"* (照鏡手法, Mandarin: ***ZHAO JING SHOU FA***, Cantonese: ***ZIU GENG SAU FAAT***) – a blocking movement with the side of the forearm from the inside to outside, in the final phase the palm is open and placed in front of your face (**Fig. 38**), **[index, p. 221]**.

[II] *"The Kitten Washes Its Muzzle"* (貓兒洗面, Mandarin: ***MAO ER XI MIAN***, Cantonese: ***MAAU JI SAI MIN***) – Scratching motion with both hands from top to bottom and towards you. One arm is slightly extended forward, and the second hand is located at the elbow of the first. Attacking the opponent's face with the "tiger's claws" while simultaneously blocking his counter-punch (**Fig. 36**), **[index, p. 221]**.

匀三又面洗兒貓

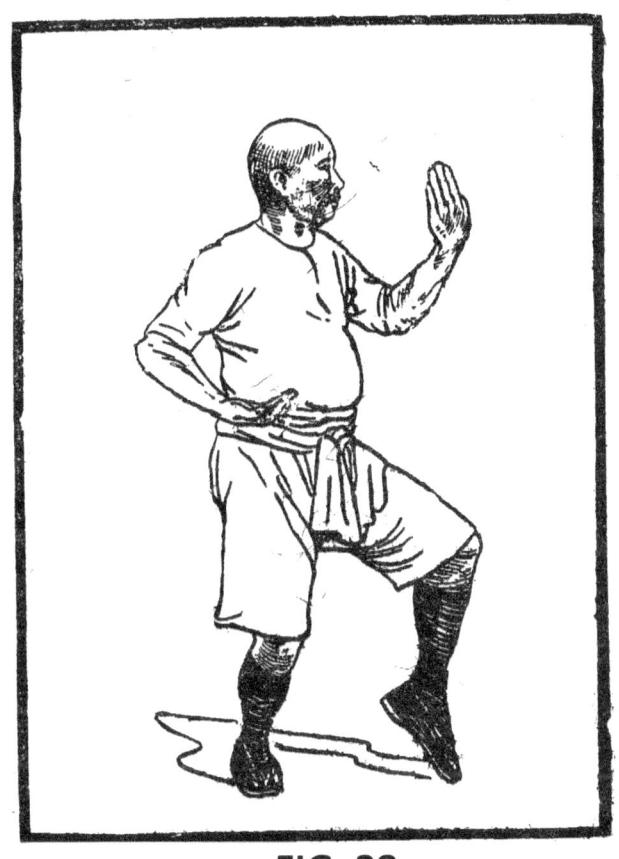

逢照鏡手法即莊頭之勢連轉貓兒洗面爪法須要倒
爪膀對胸爪對鼻連變帶馬歸槽

FIG. 38

卅九　帶馬扭身再拉後

DAI MA NU SHEN ZAI LA HOU (Mandarin)
DAAI MAA NAU SAN ZOI LAAI HAU (Cantonese)

39. To take the Horse by the Bridle, to Twist the Torso, and to Pull Back Again.

The technique "To Take the Horse by the Bridle and Bring It Back to the Stall"[I] is used if the enemy attacks with the "Overhanging Fist"[II]. I repel his attack with my arms in time, at the same time, make a grip, pull him back, and then take the stance JI NG MAA[III]. It is necessary to push forward from this position, then immediately to grip and to pull back.

Commentaries: A series of techniques to the left side (**Figs. 38, 39**) repeat similar actions in the right-side stance (**Figs. 35, 36, 37**). The only difference lies in the final position. After a blow with your two "claws," you catch the enemy's clothes and pull him to yourself. Now, unlike the previous series, you turn yourself not to 180 degrees but to 90 degrees clockwise and take the position shown in **Fig. 39** (the left leg stays on the spot, and the right leg is drawn to the left and back).

[I] *"To Take the Horse by the Bridle and Bring It Back to the Stall"* (帶馬歸槽拉, Mandarin: *DAI MA GUI CAO LA*, Cantonese: *DAAI MAA GWAI COU LAAI*) – i.e., to catch the enemy's clothes and to pull him towards yourself, at the same time to move the body back and to shift the center of gravity to the back supporting leg (Fig. 39), **[index, p. 226]**.

[II] *"Overhanging Fist"* (掛拳, Mandarin: *GUA QUAN*, Cantonese: *GWA KYUN*) - blow (or a block) with the back side of the fist and (or) the outer side of the forearm delivered from up to down. The fist moves from the shoulder level to the waist, making a semi-circle in the vertical plane **[index, p. 222]**.

[III] *JI NG MAA*, 子午馬, or *"Bow and Arrow Stance"* **[see index, p. 220]**.

帶馬扭身再拉後

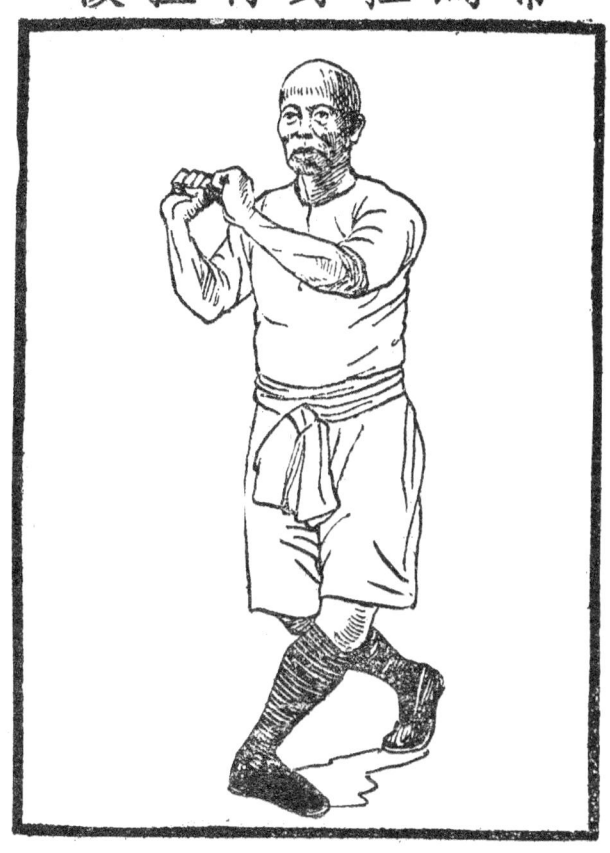

帶馬歸槽之法如敵人一掛拳打來我即用手一攻一
揸拉歸後連轉子午馬此勢須一推然後帶後

FIG. 39

四十 右脚一出子午馬

YOU JIAO YI CHU ZI WU MA (Mandarin)
JAU GEUK JAT CHEUT JI NG MAA (Cantonese)

40. Make a Step with the Right Foot, Take the Stance JI NG MAA.

Stand straight in the JI NG MAA stance, the front leg like a drawn bow, the back leg like an arrow. When the enemy attacks you with blows, one after another without a break, chop with your forearms, raise on the left, lower on the right, parry the blow, and immediately strike, using the "Paired Overhanging Fist"[I] technique. It is a diverse application of the "Hand of 1000 Characters" technique from one position.

Commentaries: From the position shown in **Fig. 39**, your right foot steps forward, and you take the position shown in **Fig. 40**. Then, without changing the stance, you carry out the technique *SEUNG CHIT BONG* (**Cut with a Pair of Wings, Fig. 41**).

[I] *"Paired Overhanging Fist"* (雙掛拳, Mandarin: *SHUANG GUA QUAN*, Cantonese: *SEUNG GWA KYUN*) - simultaneous blows (or a block) with the backsides of both fists and (or) the outer sides of forearms delivered from up to down. The fists move from the forehead level forward and down to the chest level **[see index, p. 222]**.

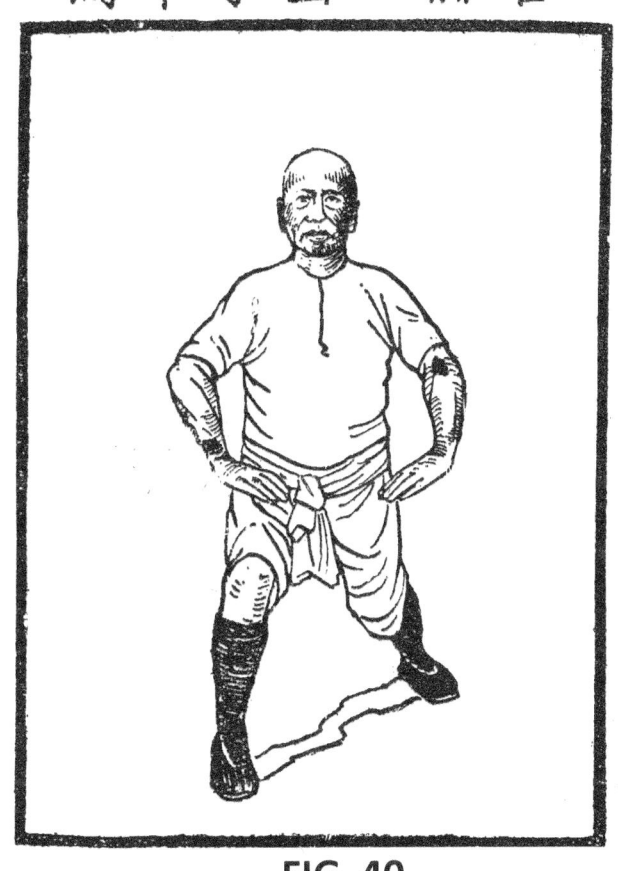

立正子午馬前弓後箭雙攻切膀左起右落一撥一割一企是為雙掛拳之法即千字一企之勢

FIG. 40

QIAN GONG HOU JIAN SHUANG QIE BANG (Mandarin)
CIN GUNG HAU ZIN SEUNG CHIT BONG (Cantonese)

41. The Bow is in Front, the Arrow is Behind, a Pair of Cutting Wings.

The technique "A Pair of Cutting Wings"[I] is used if the enemy resorts to the "Stable Gold Bridge."[II] If he "entangles" my arms and presses my elbows, I immediately employ "The Hand Breaking a Line"[III] and suppress his attack. If the enemy is discouraged and retreats, I must pursue him. Otherwise, he will not give me a chance to advance.

Commentaries: When you are in the posture shown in **Fig. 41**, change the position of your arms to the opposite: the left hand goes down, while the right hand goes up. ***"A Pair of Cutting Wings"*** means using the technique ***"The Hand Breaking a Line"*** in a fight. If the enemy tries to deliver a

---

[I] *"A Pair of Cutting Wings"* (雙切膀, Mandarin: *SHUANG QIE BANG*, Cantonese: *SEUNG CHIT BONG*) - simultaneous blocking with both arms of an enemy's attack at the upper and the middle level with using *"Arm Like a Wing"* (膀手, *BANG SHOU*), Fig.41, **[index, p. 222]**.

[II] *"Stable Gold Bridge"* (定金橋, Mandarin: ***DING JIN QIAO***, Cantonese: ***DING GAM KIU***) - the arms are extended forward at chest level, parallel to each other, but not fully straightened; elbows pointing down; four of your fingers are completely straight and spread wide with effort, the thumb is perpendicular to the palm plane and directed forward. Your wrists are bent toward the outer side of your forearms. You should feel some tension in your wrists and thumbs. This is one of the basic exercises for strengthening the forearms **(Figs. 12, 48, pp. 50, 122) [index, p. 225]**. See also Lam Sai Wing, *Iron Thread. Southern Shaolin Hung Gar Kung Fu Classics Series* (2008).

[III] *"The Hand Breaking a Line"* (破排手, Mandarin: *PO PAI SHOU*, Cantonese: *PO PAI SAU*) - circle and push blocking movements with palms and forearms, which can be performed in a vertical, horizontal, or diagonal direction **[see index, p. 218]**.

series of blows from a middle distance to you, you resolutely engage him in close-range fighting and obstruct possible directions of attacks with a cross-like movement of your arms in the front plane. When using this technique, you should act swiftly to forestall the enemy.

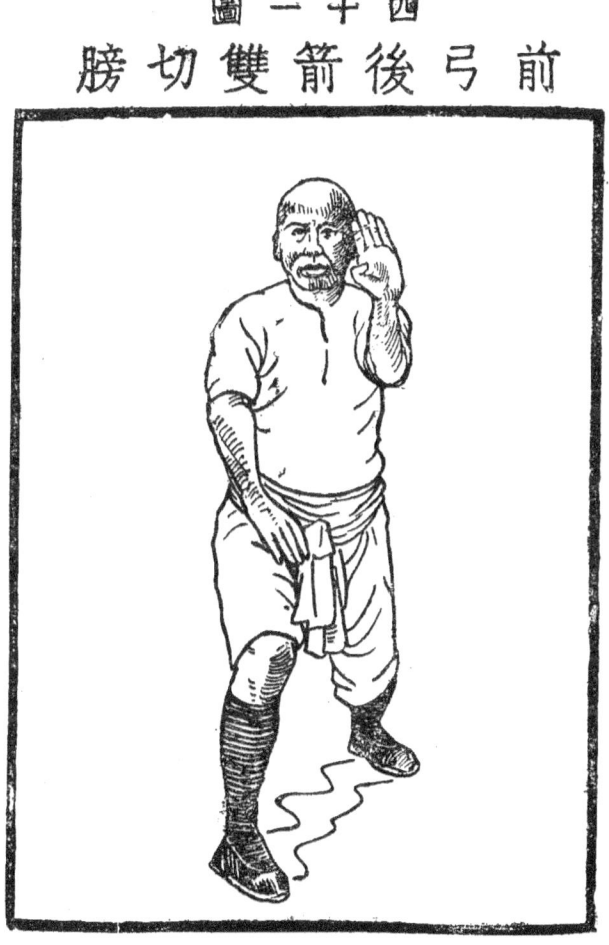

四十一圖
前弓後箭雙切膀

雙切膀手法如敵人用定金橋串我手睜我即用破排手伏之倘敵人退馬歸後再出莊頭亦不可進前

FIG. 41

四十二　左上右落千字手
ZUO SHANG YOU LUO QIAN ZI SHOU (Mandarin)
JO SOENG JAU LOK CIN ZI SAU (Cantonese)

42. To Raise on the Left, to Lower on the Right, the Hand of 1000 Characters.

Using the method of "A Hand of a Thousand Characters,"[I] you take aside, separate, and draw a straight line - this is a strike. Those are actions of "The Hand of a Thousand Characters." After separating "A Thousand Characters," you at once attack with "A Thousand Hands" - it means "to draw a line." Then, you immediately pass to the technique "Paired Overhanging Fist."[II]

Commentaries: You move your right foot backward from the position *JI NG MAA* (or "A Bow and an Arrow", **Fig. 41**) and take the position shown in **Fig. 42**. The right arm blocks an enemy's blow at a middle level. Without stopping, your right foot steps forward, and you return to the position *JI NG MAA*. At the same time, your right forearm moves from down to up and blocks a possible enemy's attack at the upper and middle levels. At the final stage, your forearm is placed horizontally at the level of your forehead, your elbow is bent, and your palm is open and directed forward. At this moment, your left arm

---

[I] *"The Hand of 1000 Characters"* (千字手, Mandarin: **QIAN ZI SHOU**, Cantonese: **CIN JI SAU**) - a wide range of blows and blocking with the arm (forearm), both from the inside out and the outside in, at different angles to the line of attack. The variations of this technique are shown in **Figs. 29, 35, 38, 42 [index, p. 219]**. See also: *Lam Sai Wing, "Tiger and Crane".*

[II] *"Paired Overhanging Fist"* (雙掛拳, Mandarin: **SHUANG GUA QUAN**, Cantonese: **SEUNG GWA KYUN**) - simultaneous blows (or a block) with the backsides of both fists and (or) the outer sides of forearms delivered from up to down. The fists move from the forehead level forward and down to the chest level **[index, p. 222]**.

delivers a blow with the fingertips of an open palm to the enemy's face or his throat. Movements of your arms and legs should be coordinated, in other words, "hands and feet come at the same time."

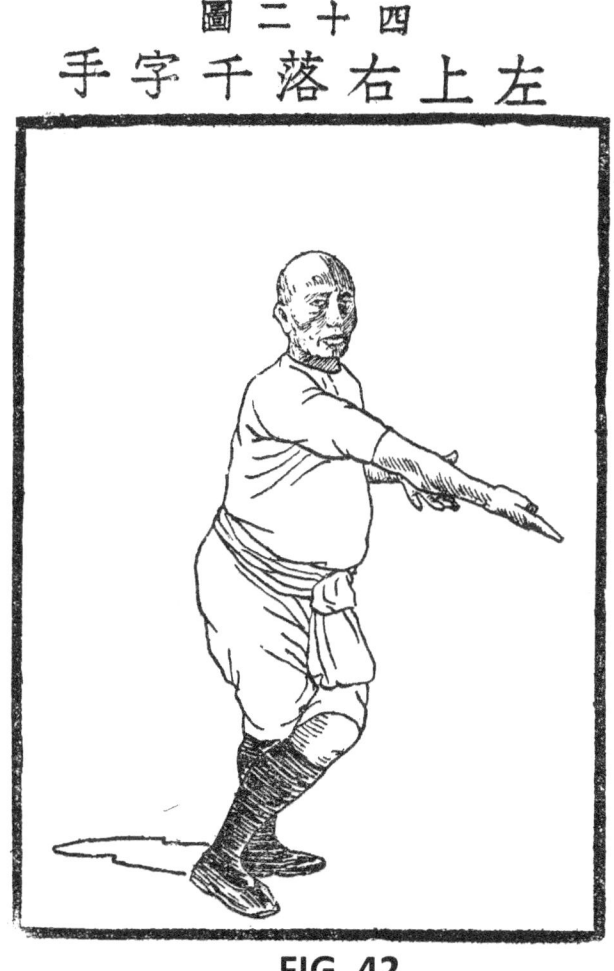

圖二十四
手字千落右上左

逢千字手法一撇手爲千字之一撇一劃爲千字之一
劃即攻千手一企爲千字中之一企即雙掛拳法

FIG. 42

四十三　拉馬抽拳雙掛落

LA MA CHOU QUAN SHUANG GUA LUO (Mandarin)
LAAI MAA CAU KYUN SEUNG GWA LOK (Cantonese)

43. Take the Horse by the Reins, Pull the Fists Towards You, Paired Overhanging Fists from Top to Bottom.

"Paired Overhanging Blows from Up to Down"[I] is used if the enemy continues with the "Double Attack with Arms Like Scissors."[II] You pull your fists towards your chest and deliver paired blows from top to bottom to the level of the waist region with both fists. If he opposes you with "A pair of wings" from the left and the right and then tries to push you away, immediately use "The Hand Breaking a Line"[III] and break his attack.

Commentaries: After delivering a blow with fingertips in the stance **JI NG MAA** ("A Bow and an Arrow"), you shift the body weight to your rear (left) leg and take **"Hanging Foot**

[I] *"Paired Overhanging Blows from Up to Down"* (掛搥雙落, Mandarin: *GUA CHUI SHUANG LUO*, Cantonese: *GWA CEOI SEUNG LOK*) - simultaneous blows (or a block) with the backsides of both fists and (or) the outer sides of forearms delivered from up to down. The fists move from the forehead level forward and down to the chest level. The same as the *"Paired Overhanging Fist"* (雙掛拳) **[index, p. 222]**.

[II] *"Double Attack with Arms Like Scissors"* (較剪雙攻手法, Mandarin: *JIAO JIAN SHUANG GONG SHOU FA*, Cantonese: *GAAU JIN SEUNG GUNG SAU FAAT*) - simultaneous blows with two arms in the horizontal plane **[see index, p. 217]**.

[III] *"The Hand Breaking a Line"* (破排手, Mandarin: *PO PAI SHOU*, Cantonese: *PO PAI SAU*) - circle and push blocking movements with palms and forearms, which can be performed in a vertical, horizontal, or diagonal direction **[see index, p. 218]**.

Stance" (or *"The Cat's Stance"*). Both hands are clenched into fists and drawn backward with a jerk at the level of your shoulders. This position is shown in **Fig. 58** (a view from the back, left-side stance). In this case, you act in the right-side stance: your posture is a mirror reflection of **Fig. 58**. Then your right foot steps forward, and you return to the stance *JI NG MAA.* When your right foot touches the ground, you deliver paired blows *Double Attack with Arms Like Scissors*. When your fists move from up to down, they make a semicircle in the vertical plane and lower to your waist.

圖三十四

落掛雙拳抽馬拉

掛撻雙落如敵人用較剪雙攻手法招之我即將手一
收再用雙拳打他腰部左右他用雙翅一推我即用破
排手破之

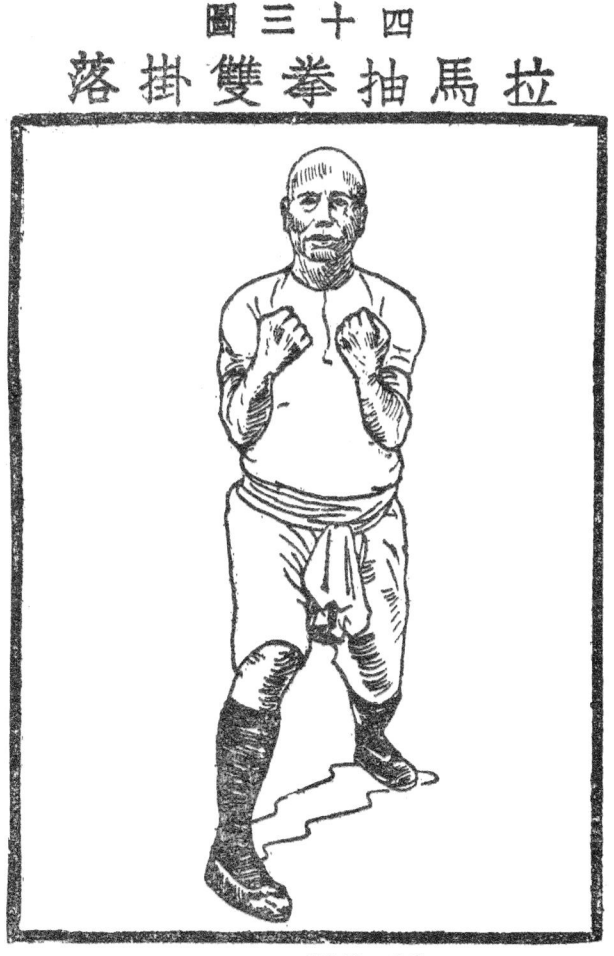

FIG. 43

四十四　進馬兜静雙虎爪

JIN MA DOU ZHENG SHUANG HU ZHAO (Mandarin)
JEON MAA DAU ZAANG SEUNG FU JAAU (Cantonese)

44. Go On in the stance JI NG MAA, Circle with the Elbow, a Pair of Tiger's Claws.

If the opponent avoids my blows and goes into a counterattack, I retreat to the position SEI PING MAA[I] and immediately switch to the technique "The Fierce Tiger Lurking Under a Rock"[II] to dodge his attack. But he approaches me, and I, without delay, deliver the blow "The Bull Strikes with Its Horn."[III] Then, I immediately go on with "The Blow that Breaches the Sky."[IV]

Commentaries: Shift the body center of gravity backward from the right side stance *JI NG MAA* (Fig. 43) and take the position *"Fierce Tiger Lurking Under a Rock"* (Fig. 44). At the same time, the right forearm makes a semicircle

---

[I] *Horse Riding Stance* (四平馬, Mandarin: *SEI PING MA*, Cantonese: *SEI PING MAA*) – literally: *"Four Levels Horse Stance"*, also known as the *"Horse Stance"* (馬步, *MA BU*) (Fig. 44), **[see index, p. 220]**.

[II] *"The Fierce Tiger Lurking Under a Rock"* (猛虎隱巖, Mandarin: *MENG HU YING YANG*, Cantonese: *MAANG FU JAN NGAAM*) – dodging an enemy attack by moving to a low *SEI PING MAA* stance with a deflecting block with the elbow and forearm (Fig. 44), **[index, p. 218]**.

[III] *"The Bull Strikes with Its Horn"* (牛角搥, Mandarin: *NIU JIAO CHUI*, Cantonese: *NGAU GOK CEOI*) – a circular punch delivered with the elbow bent (similar to a hook in boxing) (Fig. 45), **[index, p. 215]**.

[IV] *"The Blow that Breaches the Sky"* (通天搥, Mandarin: *TONG TIAN CHUI*, Cantonese: *TUNG TIN CEOI*) – punch from down to up (similar to an uppercut in boxing) **[index, p. 215]**.

movement in the vertical plane and blocks an enemy's attack to your head or your breast.

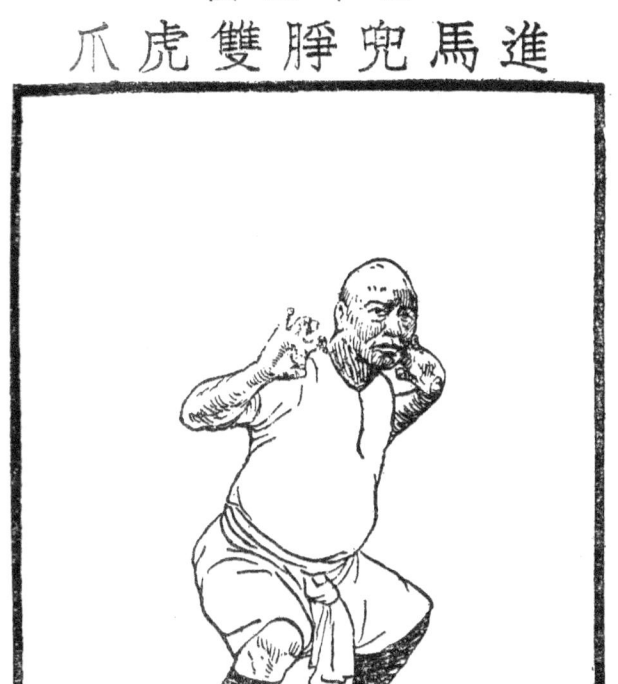

進馬兜脬雙虎爪

圖四十四

此勢若兜脬不應我即連轉猛虎隱巖之勢他入我我
即用牛角搥一搥打出連環一通天搥打他

FIG. 44

四十五　牛角一搥轉通天

NIU JIAO YI CHUI ZHUAN TONG TIAN (Mandarin)
NGAU GOK JAT CEOI JYUN TUNG TIN (Cantonese)

45. The Bull Strikes with Its Horn, Go On and Breach the Sky.

I meet the enemy with the blow "The Bull Strikes with Its Horn"[I] and hit him on the head. Then, I attack the enemy in the chin with the punch "The Blow that Breaches the Sky."[II] If the enemy parries my blows and rushes through the Small Gate[III] to try to punch or catch me, I grab and rake with my right hand and throw my left palm up. I move forward step by step and suppress the enemy. Thus, I advanced four steps in a row."

Commentaries: It is necessary to shift the body's center of gravity to the front standing leg from the position shown in **Fig. 44** , take the stance ***JI NG MAA*** ("A Bow and an Arrow"), and at the same time deliver a side blow ***"The Bull Strikes with Its Horn"*** (**Fig. 45**) to the enemy's head with your left fist. In the final phase, the arm is bent at almost 90 degrees and is located in a horizontal plane, the fist is positioned vertically, palm forward, the blow is delivered with the knuckles (**Fig. 44)**. Then, without pause, deliver a blow from down to up to his chin with your right fist. If the enemy succeeded in parrying the two of your previous blows and passes to a counterattack, pass to the technique ***"Throwing the Elbow Up"*** presented in **Fig. 46**.

[I] [see index, p. 215].

[II] [see index, p. 215].

[III] i.e., enters into close combat.

牛角一搥轉通天

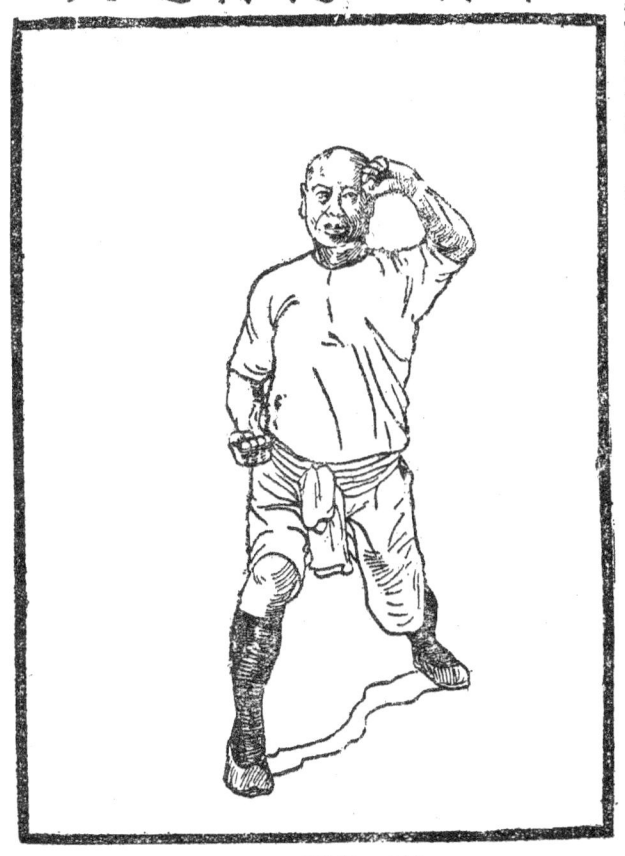

逢牛角搥須打他之頭部通天搥須打他人之下扒如
敵人由小門沖入腰部我即將右手扒左手拋掌步步
進迫連進四勻

FIG. 45

四十六　囬馬拋睜上四勻

HUI MA PAO ZHENG SHANG SI YUN (Mandarin)
WUI MAA PAAU ZAANG SOENG SEI WAN (Cantonese)

46. Turn Around the Horse, Throwing the Elbow Up Four Times.

After forwarding in the JI NG MAA stance and Throwing the Elbows Up[I], turn around and lower yourself in the SEI PING MAA stance[II]. Pull your hands to your waist and "root" in the stance. Then, raise your fists to the sides of your chest. The waist is lowered, the power is generated in the feet and controlled by the waist, the breath-Qi and the Force-Li are united. Gather all the power and cut with the forearms from top to bottom[III]. In this case, the outer sides of the forearms are used.

Commentaries: From the previous position ***JI NG MAA*** (**Fig. 45**), your right foot steps backward and to the right at a 45-degree angle. At the same time, the left hand is transformed into "tiger's claws" and makes a "raking" movement from left to right, taking a position before your breast. In the final posture, the elbow is bent, and the arm is in the horizontal plane. With this movement, you deflect aside a blow aimed at your breast or face. At the same time, you deliver a blow from down to up to the elbow bend of the enemy's attacking arm

---

[I] ***"Throwing the Elbow Up"*** (拋睜上, Mandarin: ***PAO ZHENG SHANG***, Cantonese: ***PAAU ZAANG SOENG***) – blocking (or blow) with the elbow from bottom to top, in the final phase, the arm is completely bent, the hand is located near the temple, the elbow is at the level of the chin (**Fig. 46**), **[index, p. 226]**.

[II] The following describes the actions related to **Fig. 47**.

[III] ***"Cutting with Wings"*** (切膀, Mandarin: ***QIE BANG***, Cantonese: ***CHIT BONG***) – blocking with the outer sides of the forearms with the edges of the palm from top to bottom (**Figs. 11, 47**), **[index, p. 216]**.

with your right elbow or, if the distance permits, to his breast or chin. Then your left foot steps forward and to the left at 45 45-degree angle, and you exercise the technique to the other side. All in all, four turns (and the elbow's blows) are made. It is necessary to resolutely enter the enemy's defense and deliver hard blows with your elbows using body weight.

From this position, the techniques shown in **Figs. 11 - 16** are performed again (**Figs. 47 - 51**).

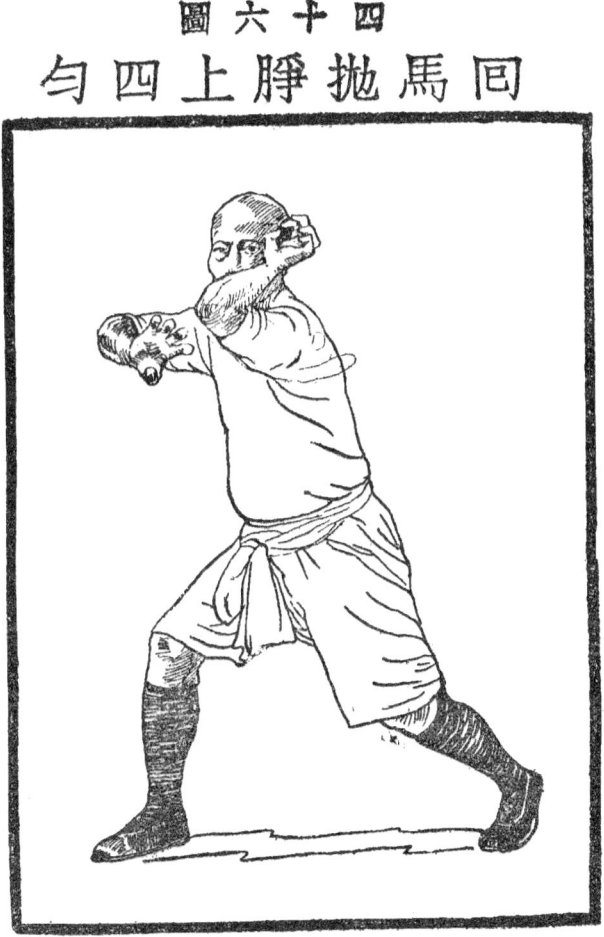

圖六十四

勻四上胛拋馬回

進馬拋胛之後轉身落正四平大馬此勢必要插腰落
馬抽拳在胸側運足氣力切膀一落即外膀之法

FIG. 46

四十七　轉身向後四平馬

ZHUAN SHEN XIANG HOU SEI PING MA (Mandarin)
JYUN SAN HOENG HAU SEI PING MAA (Cantonese)

47. Turn Around, Stand in the SEI PING MAA Position.

If the enemy delivers a blow, put your palms together and deflect a blow aside. Then, with your hands in the position "One Finger" (JAT ZI) you continuously push, than "Pull" (抽, CAU), "Cut" (割, GOT), "Catch" (揸, ZA), and "Divide" (分, FAN) - all those movements are done in succession.

Commentaries: After striking four times with your elbows, turn to 180 degrees and take the *JI NG MAA* stance (**Fig. 47**). Thus, you face the initial point from which you started the Taolu (form). Actions shown in **Figs. 47-51** coincide entirely with actions shown in **Figs. 11-16**. The author names them in succession in the text to this picture.

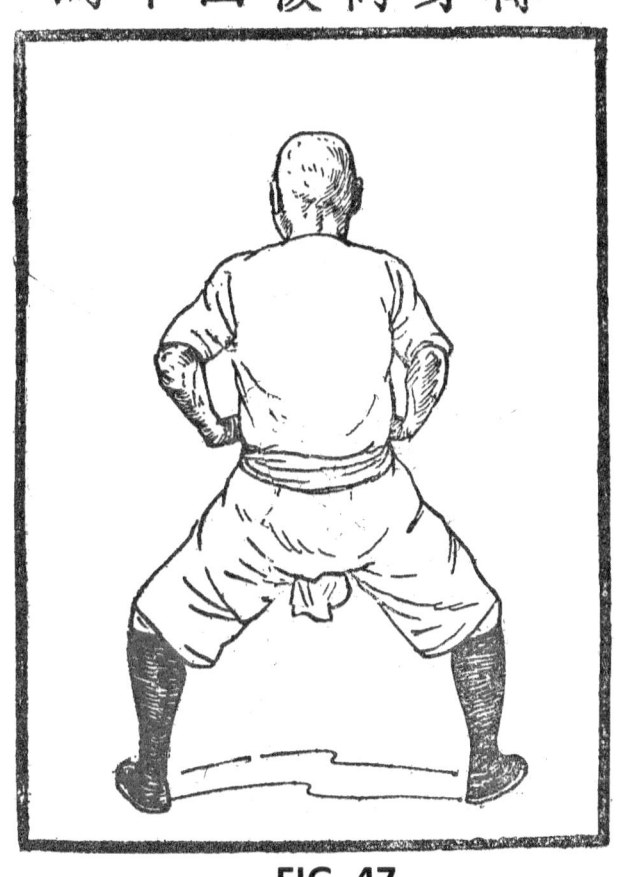

FIG. 47

如敵人一拳打來我用合掌分開轉一指手連抹之抹一抽一劃一揸一分之勢

四十八　雙膀切落合掌分

SHUANG BANG QIE LUO HE ZHANG FEN (Mandarin)
SEUNG BONG CHIT LOK HAP JEUNG FAN (Cantonese)

48. Cut with Both Arms by Lowering Them; Join the Palms, Then Bring Them Apart.

After performing the technique "Paired Arms like Wings", place your palms together, then spread them apart into the "Flying Crane"[I] position. There are the following "Crane" techniques: "A Crane Wing,"[II] "A Crane Beak,"[III] "A Well-Fed Crane,"[IV] "A Hungry Crane."[V] There is also the stance "A Single Leg Flying Crane."[VI]

Commentaries: A series of techniques named in the title is shown in **Figs. 10-12**. The posture "A flying Crane" refers to the technique ***DING GAM KIU*** - the ***"Stable Gold Bridge"[VII]***. This position is illustrated in **Fig. 48**. Other

---

[I] *"A Flying Crane"* (飛鶴, Mandarin: **FEI HE**, Cantonese: **FEI HOK**).

[II] *"A Crane Wing"* (鶴翅, Mandarin: **HE CHI**, Cantonese: **HOK CHI**).

[III] *"A Crane Beak"* (鶴頂, Mandarin: **HE DING**, Cantonese: **HOK DENG**).

[IV] *"A Well-Fed Crane"* (飽鶴, Mandarin: **BAO HE**, Cantonese: **BAAU HOK**).

[V] *"A Hungry Crane"* (餓鶴, Mandarin: **E HE**, Cantonese: **NGO HOK**).

[VI] *"Single Leg Flying Crane"* (獨脚飛鶴, Mandarin: **DU JIAO FEI HE**, Cantonese: **DUK GEUK FEI HOK**).

[VII] *"Stable Gold Bridge"* (定金橋, Mandarin: **DING JIN QIAO**, Cantonese: **DING GAM KIU**) - the arms are extended forward at chest level, parallel to each other, but not fully straightened; elbows pointing down; four of your fingers are completely straight and spread wide with effort, the thumb is perpendicular to the palm plane and directed forward. Your wrists are bent

techniques mentioned here do not belong to this *TAO*; however, they can often be found in the book by Lam Sai Wing **"Tiger and Crane."**

圖八十四
分掌合落切膀雙

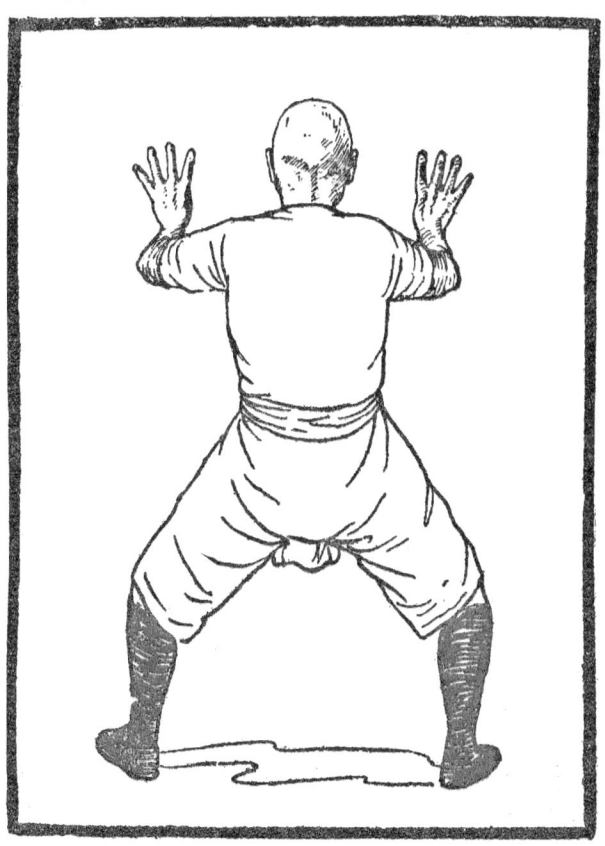

雙膀手法合掌一分即飛鶴之勢鶴有鶴翅鶴頂飽鶴

餓鶴獨脚飛鶴之勢

FIG. 48

---

toward the outer side of your forearms. You should feel some tension in your wrists and thumbs. This is one of the basic exercises for strengthening the forearms **(Figs. 12, 48, pp. 50, 122) [index, p. 225]**. See also Lam Sai Wing, *Iron Thread. Southern Shaolin Hung Gar Kung Fu Classics Series* (2008).

四十九　一指撑天三株出
YI ZHI CHENG TIAN SAN ZHU CHU (Mandarin)
JAT ZI CAANG TIN SAAM ZYU CHEUT (Cantonese)

49. Support the Sky with One Finger, Perform the "Three Openings"[I].

This is a Hung Gar technique. Raise one finger up and push three times with tension. Direct the force into the arms and "bridges" (forearms) and push three times with tension. Then throw the elbows, pierce with the hands, spread, pull, cut, grab. Due to this, you train the strength of your "bridges" (forearms).

Commentaries: Here, the techniques shown in **Figs. 47-51** are named in succession. As noted above, they coincide entirely with the actions shown in **Figs. 11-16**.

[I] *"Three Openings"* (三株, Mandarin: *SAN ZHU*, Cantonese: *SAAM ZYU*) is one of the most important basic techniques of *Hung Gar* style inherited from the *Southern Shaolin*. The *Shaolin "Treatises on Fighting Arts"* say: *"It is necessary to pay special attention to the fact that the Mind would guide the Breath-Qi and the Breath-Qi should act in unity with the physical Force-Li. The Breath-Qi must strengthen the physical Force-Li and the Force-Li must guide the Breath-Qi"*. This, in outward appearance, a simple exercise, is aimed at training the said cooperation. The hands are in a position of *"One Finger"* (*JAT ZI*), as shown in **Fig. 13**. The initial position: the palms are on the shoulder level, and the elbows are lowered on the sides. Take a sharp breath in through the mouth and "close" *Qi* (strain your stomach and hold breathing), then slowly, with an effort, pull the palms aside on the shoulder level **[index, p. 225]**.

一指撐天三株出

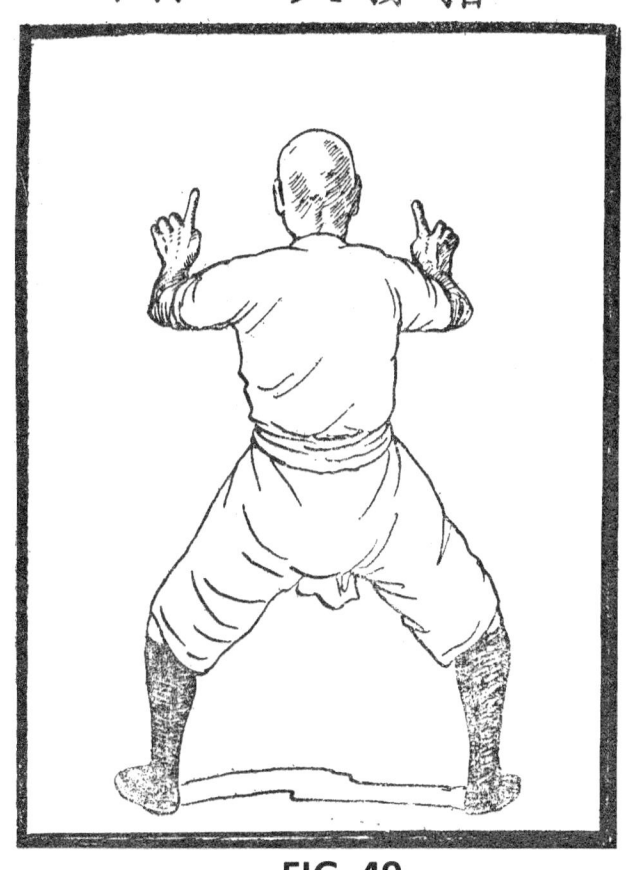

洪拳之法一指三株以運力在手橋之內三株之後一
拋胂一標串手一定一抽一割一揸一分以練橋力

FIG. 49

五十　標串手法定金橋

BIAO CHUAN SHOU FA DING JIN QIAO (Mandarin)
BIU CYUN SAU FAAT DING GAM KIU (Cantonese)

50. The Method "Do a Mark with a Piercing Hand", and Stable Golden Bridge.

BIU CYUN SAU [I] is a method of continuous execution of the technique "Piercing Hand". If the enemy covers my palm, I also do a covering movement that continuously transforms into a "piercing" blow. These are piercing strikes from the Snake style. If the enemy uses this technique against me, I enter the Small Gate [II], employ the technique "Three-Star Hook Spring Leg" [III], and break his attack.

Commentaries: Fig. 50 shows a double blow ***BIU CYUN SAU*** (back view). The decisive factor of the employment of ***BIU CYUN SAU*** in a fight as a continuous series of blows is speed. One must act swiftly, like a biting snake, and deliver strikes to vulnerable points of the enemy. Strikes follow in

---

[I] **"Do a Mark with a Piercing Hand"** (標串掌, Mandarin: **BIAO CHUAN ZHANG**, Cantonese: **BIU CYUN JEUNG**) - a thrust blow with the ends of fingers of an open palm **[see index, p. 217]**.

[II] **"Enter the Small Gate"** means to attack the enemy at a lower level. The theory of the **Hung Gar** style identifies five directions of attack, or five **"Gates"** (門, Cantonese: **MUN**), through which one can enter the enemy's defense space. Those are the upper, lower, and middle levels, as well as the left and right sides **[index, p. 217]**.

[III] **"Three-Star Hook Spring Leg"** (三星鉤彈腳, Mandarin: **SAN XING ZHU TAN JIAO**, Cantonese: **SAAM SING KAU TAAN GEUK**) - a low sweeping kick with the shin (lower shinbone), hooking and sweeping of the front-standing leg of the enemy, followed by a kick to the knee or ankle of his supporting leg or a reverse leg sweep **[see index, p. 226]**.

succession to stun the enemy and not to give him a chance to re-form for a counterattack.

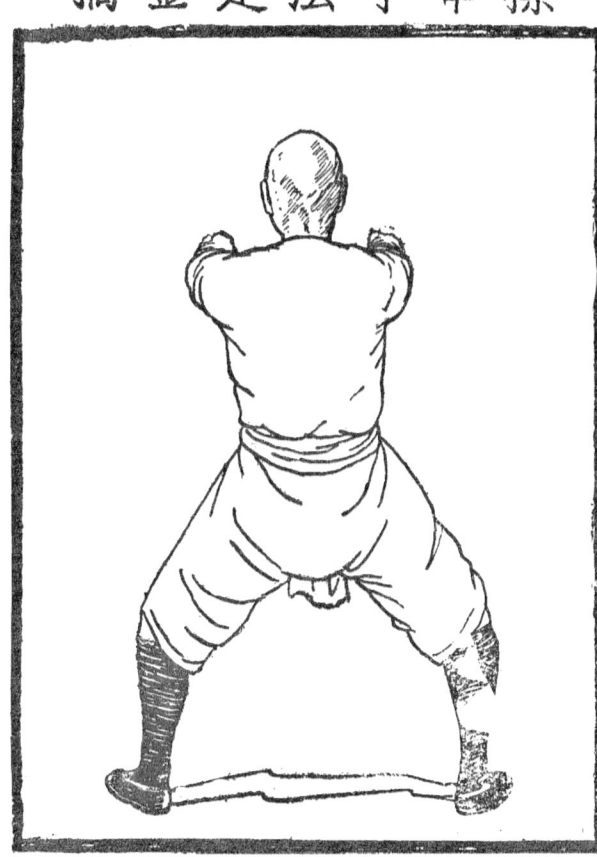

五 十 圖
標 串 手 法 定 金 橋

此法連環標串他人如我掌我亦用連環如串手法即
蛇形手法一般倘敵人用此法攻我我必要由小門用
三星抝彈脚法破之

FIG. 50

五十一 雙抽雙割一揸分

SHUANG CHOU SHUANG GE YI ZHA FEN (Mandarin)
SEUNG CAU SEUNG GOT JAT ZA FAN (Cantonese)

51. Both Pull Out and Both Cut, Grasp and Bring Apart.

To achieve the right "Paired Gold Bridge," the hands should be in the "Four Fingers Support the Sky"[I] position. In this posture, you should direct force to the fingertips. Then pull your hands apart and cut with your forearms. This is called "A Cutting Bridge"[II]. If the enemy attacks you with "A Rising Bridge", you immediately oppose with the "Cutting Bridge"[III] technique to "cut" his attacking arm, and you will surely win.

Commentaries: Here, the use of ***"A Cutting Bridge"*** is described. Pay attention that the same movement that has another name ***"Dividing the Gold Bridge"*** is shown in **Fig. 16.** There are frequent cases in the traditional Kung Fu when movements that seem to be almost identical have different names. It corresponds to many variants of the combat use of those movements. In this case, ***"Dividing the Gold Bridge"***

[I] **"Four Fingers Support the Sky"** (四指撐天, Mandarin: **SI ZHI CHENG TIAN**, Cantonese: **SEI ZI CAANG TIN**) - four of your fingers are completely straight and spread wide with effort, the thumb is perpendicular to the palm plane and directed forward. Your wrists are bent toward the outer side of your forearms. You should feel some tension in your wrists, thumbs, and fingers. This is one of the basic exercises for strengthening hands, fingers and forearms **[index, p. 218]**.

[II] **"A Cutting Bridge"** (割橋, Mandarin: **GE QIAO**, Cantonese: **GOT KIU**) - a block (or blow) using the forearm; one of the fighting applications of the **"Stable Golden Bridge"** (定金橋) technique **[index p. 216]**.

[III] **"A Rising Bridge"** (提橋, Mandarin: **TI QIAO**, Cantonese: **TAI KIU**) - a blow with the outside or side of the forearm (or fist), directed from the bottom up **[index, p. 224]**.

(**Fig. 16)** means a blow with the back side of a fist to the enemy's ribs, and the **"A Cutting Bridge"** (**Fig. 51)** means a block with the outer side of the forearm.

圖一十五
分揸一割雙抽雙

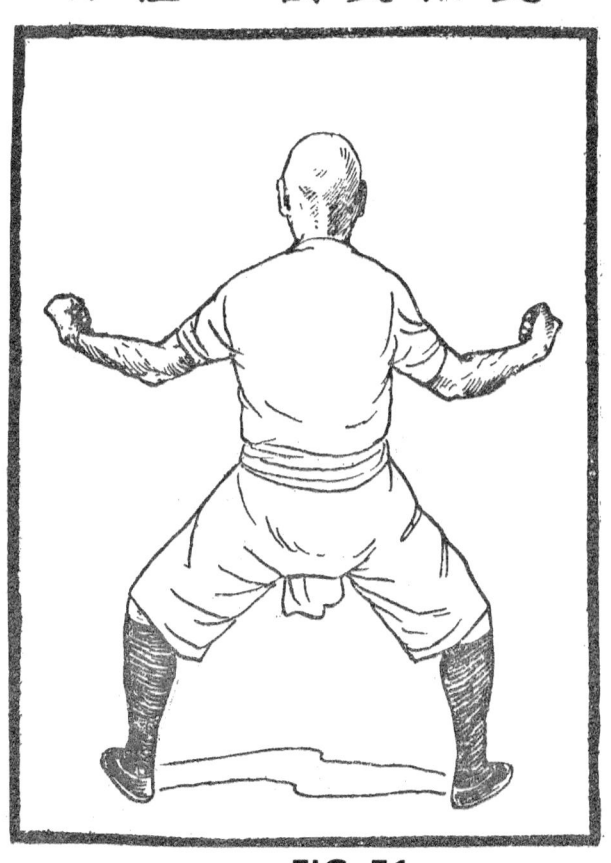

金橋雙定之法須用四指撐天然後指尾有力連將兩
手抽開一割此割橋如敵人用提橋一攻我即用割橋
一割他手必勝

FIG. 51

五十二　蝶掌一迫分漏手

DIE ZHANG YI PO FEN LOU SHOU (Mandarin)
DIP JEUNG JAT BIK FAN LAU SAU (Cantonese)

52. The Palms like Butterflies: Push and Divide, Penetrate with Hands.

If the enemy attacks me with the use of the technique "Palms like Butterflies,"[I] I can also use the "Palms like Butterflies" to oppose him. So, I repulse the "Palms like Butterflies" with the use of the "Palms like Butterflies." Even if the enemy is stronger than I, I can successfully use the technique "Penetrate with Hands"[II] and attack him.

Commentaries: You make a step forward with your right foot, turn to the left to 90 degrees, and take the **"Hanging Foot Stance"** (or *"The Cat's Stance"*). Your arms are in the position shown in **Fig. 63** (the only difference: in this case, you are in the left stance). That is the initial position for executing the technique **"Palms like Butterflies."** Your left foot makes a step forward, you take the stance **JI NG MAA** (or *"The Bow and the Arrow"*) and deliver a double palm blow (**Fig. 52**). The combat use of the **"Palms like Butterflies"** against the same technique used by the enemy is described in the commentaries to **Fig. 9**.

[I] **"Palms like Butterflies"** (蝶掌, Mandarin: **DIE ZHANG**, Cantonese: **DIP JEUNG**) - circular block with both palms in the frontal plane, followed by a simultaneous blow with open palms at two levels, the fingers of the upper palm are directed upwards, the fingers of the lower palm are directed downwards **[see index, p. 223]**.

[II] **"Turn and Divide, Penetrate with Hands"** (轉分漏手, Mandarin: **ZHUANG FEN LOU SHOU**, Cantonese: **JYUN FAN LAU SAU**) - see commentaries on **page 44**, **[see index, p. 227]**.

蝶掌一迫分漏手

五十二圖

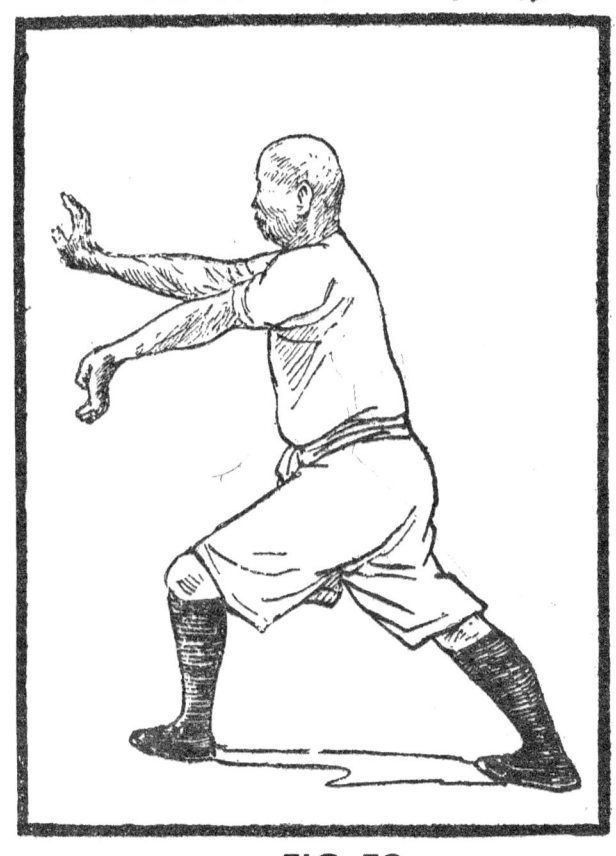

倘敵人用蝶掌先打來我亦可以用蝶掌招之此即以蝶掌破蝶掌之法如他力大我即用分漏手法攻之

FIG. 52

五十三　再攋蝶掌迫分漏

ZAI LA DIE ZHANG PO FEN LOU (Mandarin)
ZOI LAAP DIP JEUNG BIK FAN LAU (Cantonese)…

53. The Palms like Butterflies Once More, Push, Divide and Penetrate.

The enemy attacks me with a punch. I retreat to the "Hanging Foot Stance", use the "Tiger's Claws" and protect myself against his blow. If he is close to me, I attack with the "claws"[1]. Then I use the technique "Penetrate with Hands" followed by the kick. He tries to catch my leg, but my kick is like an arrow from a bow, and I hit his lower part.

Commentaries: From the position shown in **Fig. 52,** you turn on your left foot to 180 degrees clockwise and take the ***"Hanging Foot Stance."*** At the same time, you deflect with your right forearm an enemy's blow aimed at your head or your breast aside, and push his attacking arm with your left palm to the region of his elbow. The turns of your body and arm movements are done simultaneously. Your hands are in the position "claws". The final position is shown in **Fig. 63** . Then, change the hands' position with a circular movement in the front plane (the left "claws" are near the waist, the right "claws" are near the left shoulder). This is the technique ***"Turn and Divide, Penetrate with Hands"*** (***JYUN FAN LAU SAU***). Then, your right foot makes a step forward, you take the stance ***JI NG MAA*** (*"The Bow and the Arrow"*). At the same time, deliver a double blow with the ***"Palms like Butterflies"*:** the right palm is located on top, the left one is located below. Without stopping, deliver a straight kick with the heel of the left foot to the enemy's groin or his stomach. If the enemy deflects your kick aside with a sweeping movement or tries to

---

[1] This refers to blocking and attacking with the ***Tiger Claw*** at the same time, in one continuous movement.

grab your leg, sharply pull the left foot to your right knee and immediately attack the knee, shin, or instep of the enemy's front leg. The kick is delivered with the side of the foot. Then turn your torso to the right, put your left leg back, and take the stance *JI NG MAA*. Your arms are in the position shown in **Fig. 53** - this is the technique *CIN GEI* ("Entwining Skill") - see commentaries to **Fig. 54.**

圖三十五

漏分迫掌蝶撤再

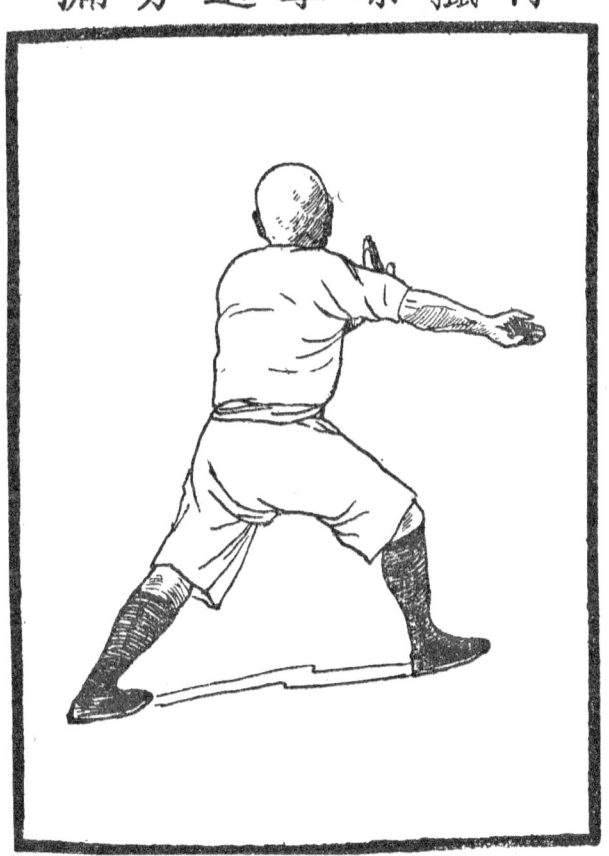

敵人用拳打來我即用吊腳單虎爪防他他近我爪我
再用分漏手連起腳攻他他用手兜我腳我即變彈弓
腳踢他下部

FIG. 53

五十四　擸掌連環拘彈脚

LA ZHANG LIAN HUAN JU TAN JIAO (Mandarin)
LAAP JEUNG LIN WAAN KEOI TAAN GEUK (Cantonese)

54. Hook with the Palm, Without Stopping Continue with the Sweeping Foot.

If the enemy is in the position SEI PING MA[I] attacks me with the "Pulling Arrow Fist"[II], I immediately answer with the technique "Entwining Skill"[III], to hook and to knock him down with the "Sweeping Foot"[IV]. If the enemy avoids my sweep by lifting his leg up and tries to kick me from above, I immediately deflect his blow aside and, without giving him time to collect himself, continue the attack. This is the "Crosswind Shakes the Willow"[V] technique.

[I] *Horse Riding Stance* (四平馬), **[see index, p. 220]**.

[II] *"Pulling Arrow Fist"* (猛箭拳, Mandarin: *MENG JIAN QUAN*, Cantonese: *MANG JIN KYUN*), full name: *"Draw the Bow and Shoot the Arrow"* (猛弓射箭, Mandarin: *MENG GONG SHE JIAN*, Cantonese: *MANG GUNG SE JIN*) - see text and commentaries to **Fig. 83**, **[index, p. 223]**.

[III] *"Entwining Skill"* (纏技, Mandarin: *CHAN JI*, Cantonese: *CIN GEI*) - deflecting block against a kick (**Fig. 53**), **[index, p. 217]**.

[IV] *"Three-Star Hook Spring Leg"* (三星鉤彈腳, Mandarin: *SAN XING ZHU TAN JIAO*, Cantonese: *SAAM SING KAU TAAN GEUK*) - a low sweeping kick with the shin (lower shinbone), hooking and sweeping of the front-standing leg of the enemy, followed by a kick to the knee or ankle of his supporting leg or a reverse leg sweep **[see index, p. 226]**.

[V] *"Crosswind Shakes the Willow"* (斜風擺柳, Mandarin: *XIE FENG BAI LIU*, Cantonese: *CE FUNG BAAI LAU*) - A sweep of the enemy's leg (or both legs) with a wide circular motion of the foot. Both arms move in the opposite direction, towards the sweeping leg, enhancing the sweeping effect (**Fig. 54**), **[index, p. 216]**.

Commentaries: The posture *"Entwining Skill"* (**Fig. 53**) is a deflecting block against a leg attack. Then turn to the right on your right foot and take the posture shown in **Fig. 54**. At the same time, do an undercutting kick with your left shin at the lower level. Your arms move in the opposite direction, i.e., from right to left. That is the ***Crosswind Shakes the Willow.***

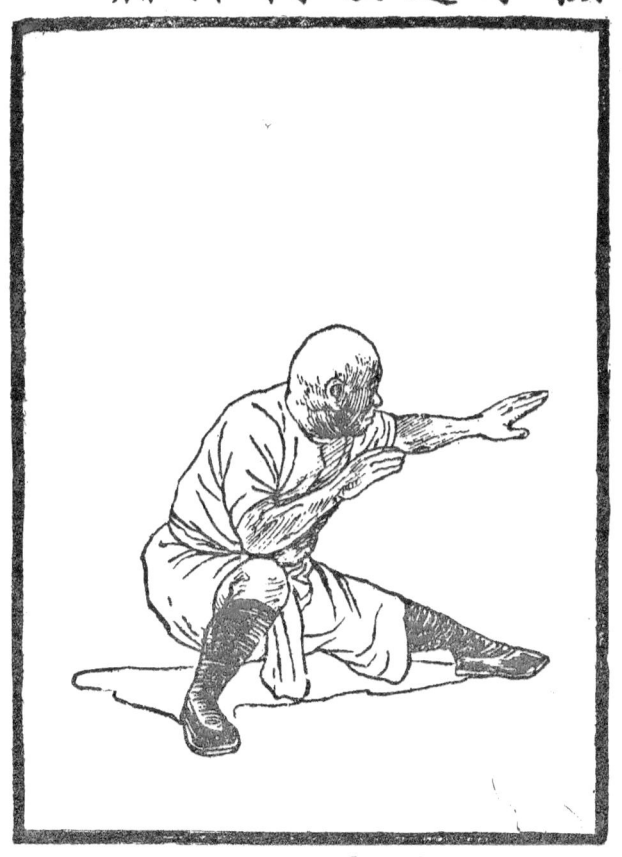

五十四圖

撳掌連環拘彈脚

如敵人落四平馬用搖箭拳打來我即用纏枝拘彈脚
法他若將先鋒脚一起我即拘他不應我即車身連轉
斜風擺柳之法

FIG. 54

五十五　斜風擺柳轉車身

XIE FENG BAI LIU ZHUAN CHE SHEN (Mandarin)
CE FUNG BAAI LAU JYUN CE SAN (Cantonese)

55. Crosswind Shakes the Willow, Turn Around.

If, during my sweeping action, Crosswind Shakes the Willow, the enemy lifts his foot and avoids my sweep, I must not continue the method. To avoid being hit, I turn around and retreat to the JI NG MAA stance. I use a Pair of Wings Cut as Knives[I], blocking at the waist level, as if I were stabbing two knives from top to bottom, precisely at the moment of landing in the JI NG MAA stance. If the opponent approaches me, I lift on the left and chop on the right.

Commentaries: If your opponent has dodged your sweep, you are in a dangerous situation, as he can deliver a powerful blow from above. Take two steps back, turning 360 degrees clockwise, and assume the left-handed ***JI NG MAA*** (or *"The Bow and the Arrow"*) stance. At the moment of landing in the stance, perform a double block ***"Pair of Wings Cut as Knives"*** (Fig. 55).

Note: Here, the series of techniques shown in **Fig. 40-45** is performed in the other direction (i.e., turning 180 degrees), and in a left-handed stance. **Figs. 55-60** show some positions from that series that were not shown in **Figs. 40-45**.

[I] ***"Pair of Wings Cut as Knives"*** (雙膀插, Mandarin: ***SHUANG BANG CHA***, Cantonese: ***SEUNG BONG CAAP***) - a block with two arms, from top to bottom, against a blow to the lower part of the body (**Fig. 55 - rear view, Fig. 40 - front view**), **[index, p. 222]**.

斜風擺柳轉車身
圖五十五

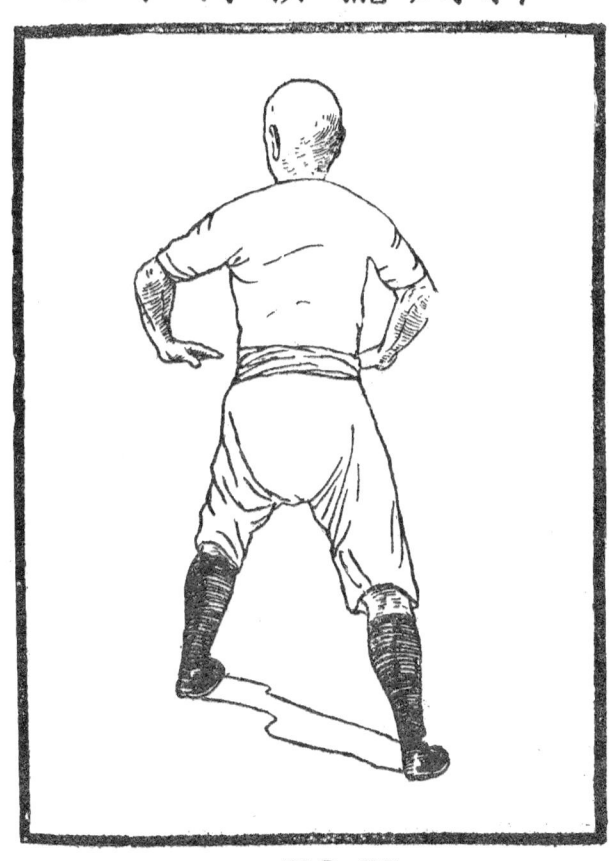

FIG. 55

逢用扚彈腳法敵人起腳扚之不應連車身敗馬子午雙膀插腰落馬倘敵人入我我即用左挑右劈招之

五十六　雙膀切落起左右
SHUANG BANG QIE LUO QI ZUO YOU (Mandarin)
SEUNG BONG CHIT LOK HEI JO JAU (Cantonese)

56. Pair of Cutting Wings, Lower and Raise on the Left and the Right.

The Pair of Cutting Wings[I] technique can beat off even a deadly "Leopard Fist"[II]. If the enemy uses the right "bridge" in the right stance MAA and tries to "pierce" me with the strike, I immediately use the "Chopping Arm" technique and block his attack. The opponent continues to attack with the "Lock the Iron Gate with a Bolt Weighing 1000 Jin"[III] technique. In response, I use the "Hand of 1000 Characters"[IV]

[I] *"A Pair of Cutting Wings"* (雙切膀, Mandarin: *SHUANG QIE BANG*, Cantonese: *SEUNG CHIT BONG*) - simultaneous blocking with both arms of an enemy's attack at the upper and the middle level with using *"Arm Like a Wing"* (膀手, *BANG SHOU*), Figs.41, 56, **[index, p. 222]**.

[II] *"Leopard Fist"* (豹拳, Mandarin: *BAO QUAN*, Cantonese: *PAAU KYUN*) - the four fingers are bent at the first phalangeal joint to expose the fore-knuckles as the striking surface, rather than the knuckles; the thumb is tucked closely against the side of the hand, **[index, p. 221]**.

[III] *"Lock the Iron Gate with a Bolt Weighing 1000 Jin"* (鐵門閂槌千斤, Mandarin: *TIE MEN SHUAN CHUI QIAN JIN*, Cantonese: - *TIT MUN SAAN CHEUI CIN GAN*) - a technique that has various applications, which are described later in this book (see **Fig. 82**), as well as in **Lam Sai Wing's** book **"Tiger and Crane"**. In this case, it refers to a simultaneous punch with both fists, from the bottom up, with an upward movement, aimed at the opponent's stomach and neck (or chin). *Jin* (Cantonese: *Gan*, 斤) is a traditional Chinese unit for weight. One *Jin* is approximately equal to 1.316 *lb* (600 *g.*) **[index, p. 221]**.

[IV] *"The Hand of 1000 Characters"* (千字手, Mandarin: *QIAN ZI SHOU*, Cantonese: *CIN JI SAU*) - a wide range of blows and blocking with the arm (forearm), both from the inside out and the outside in, at different angles to the line of attack. The variations of this technique are shown in **Figs. 29, 35, 38, 42 [see index, p. 219]**. See also: Lam Sai Wing, *"Tiger and Crane"*.

method and block his strike, sweeping it away with a diagonal movement from top to bottom.

Commentaries: see commentaries to **Fig. 40.**

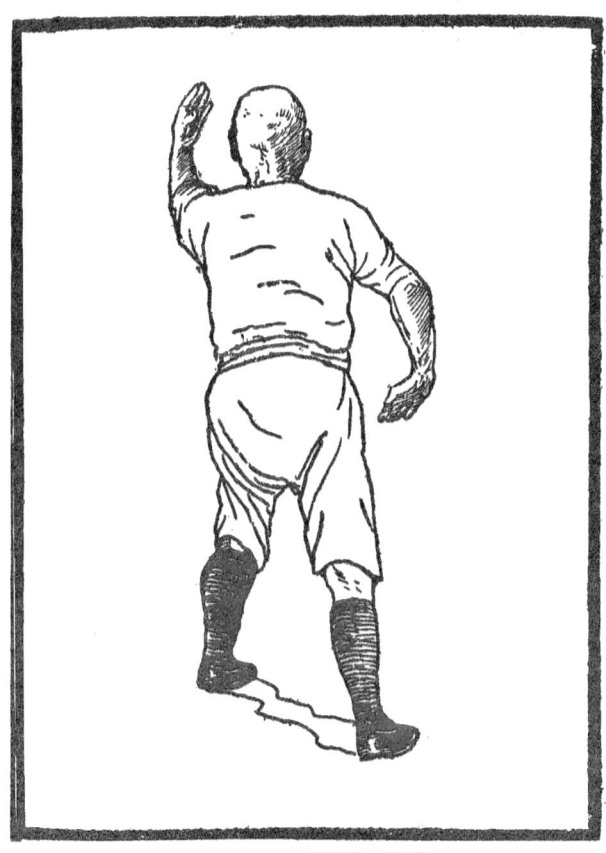

五十六圖

雙膀切落起左右

雙膀切落能破磨豹拳敵人用右橋右馬羌子拳標來
我即用兜劈手法招之敵人連轉千斤墜鐵門閂鏟來
我即用千字手法搬之

FIG. 56

五十七 一撇一劃千字手

YI PE YI HUA QIAN ZI SHOU (Mandarin)
JAT PIT JAT WAAK CIN JI SAU (Cantonese)

57. The Hand of 1000 Characters: Deflect With One Hand, Delimitate With Another One.

If the enemy attacks me in the middle section of my body, I immediately retreat to the "Hanging Foot Stance"[I] and beat off his attack with the use of "The Hand of 1000 Characters"[II]. He immediately repeats the attack, aiming the blow at my head. I use the "Chopping Arm" to frustrate his attack. That is the "Paired Work of 1000 Characters"[III].

Commentaries: see commentaries to **Fig. 42.**

[I] **"Hanging Foot Stance"** (馬吊腳, Mandarin: **MA DIAO JIAO**, Cantonese: **MAA DIU GEUK**) - known in modern *WUSHU* as the **"Cat's Stance"** (**Fig. 26**). The term **"MAA"** is used in the meaning "a stance" here **[index p. 219]**.

[II] See **Fig. 56**, **[index, p. 219]**.

[III] **"Paired Work of 1000 Characters"** (雙工千字, Mandarin: **SHUANG GONG QIAN ZI**, Cantonese: **SEUNG GUNG CHIN JI**) - Simultaneous action with both arms: one arm blocks the opponent's strike at the top level with a bottom-up movement, the other hand blocks (or strikes) at the middle level with a horizontal movement (**Fig. 57**) **[see index, p. 222]**.

五十七圖
一撇一劃千字手

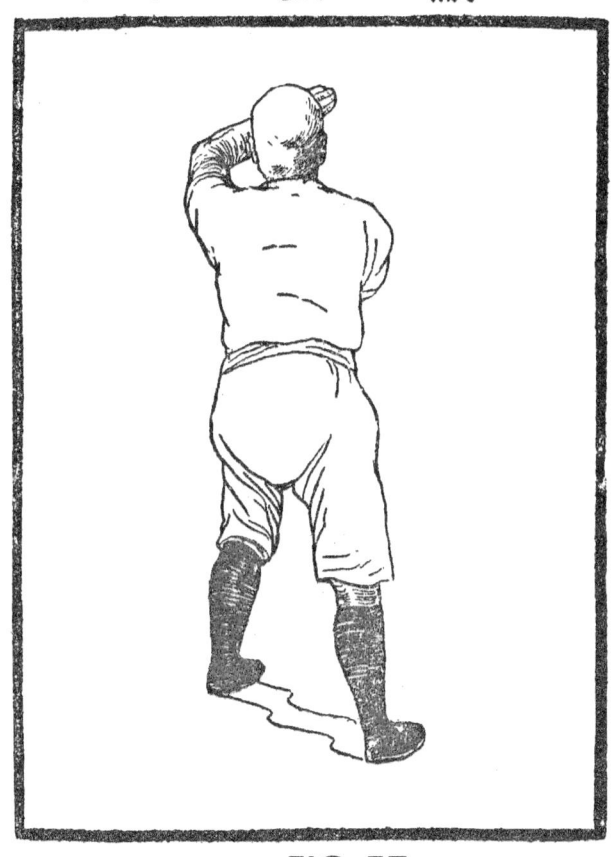

FIG. 57

如敵人由中部打來我卽用吊脚千字手撇之他再由頭部打來我用攻劈手法破之卽雙工千字之勢

五十八　拉馬抽拳雙掛落

LA MA CHOU QUAN SHUANG GUA LUO (Mandarin)
LAAI MAA CAU KYUN SEUNG GWA LOK (Cantonese)

58. Take the Horse by the Reins, Pull the Fists Towards You, Paired Hanging Fists from Top to Bottom.

When you deliver a Paired Overhanging Blow[I] with both fists, your fists should not be positioned wide (far apart). You must strike from above. If your fists are too far apart, the strike will hit the enemy's shoulders or arms and will not cause severe damage. However, if you join your fists and strike while landing in the stance, you can strike on his face, directly downwards, on his breast, heart, or other parts of the body.

Commentaries: The technique of the blow is described in the commentaries to **Fig. 43**. Here, the author describes some crucial nuances.

[I] *"Paired Overhanging Fist"* (雙掛拳, Mandarin: *SHUANG GUA QUAN*, Cantonese: *SEUNG GWA KYUN*) - simultaneous blows (or a block) with the backsides of both fists and (or) the outer sides of forearms delivered from up to down. The fists move from the forehead level forward and down to the chest level [see index, p. 222].

五十八圖
拉馬抽拳雙掛落

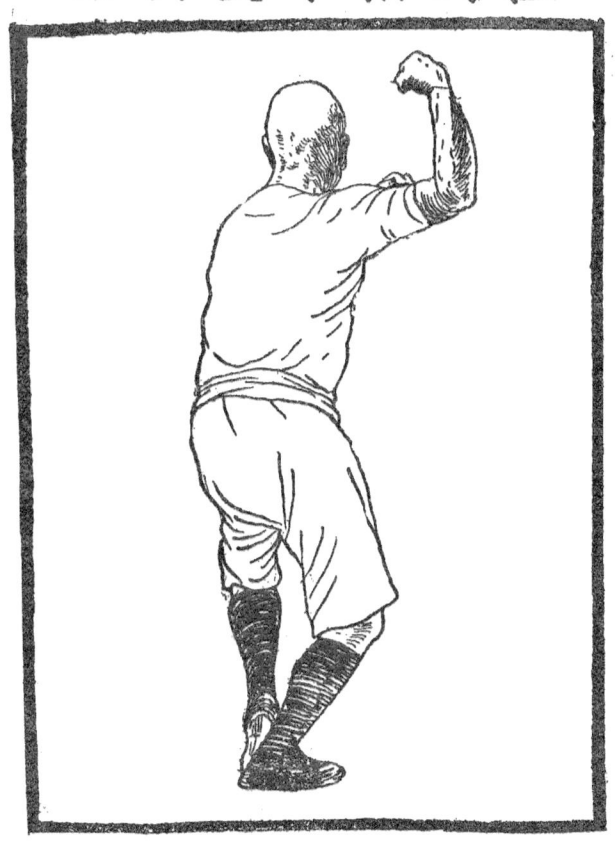

FIG. 58

逢掛拳之法雙拳不可離開掛落倘離開打落即打敵
人之肩膊不能傷他若合拳打落即可傷他面門直下
心胸等部

五十九　進馬兜掙雙虎爪

JIN MA DOU ZHENG SHUANG HU ZHAO (Mandarin)
JEON MAA DAU ZAANG SEUNG FU JAAU (Cantonese)

59. Go On in the stance MAA, Circle with the Elbow, Pair of Tiger's Claws.

The Tiger Claw techniques are listed here: "Tiger Descends from the Mountain"[I], "Single Tiger Claw"[II], "Double Tiger Claw"[III], "Black Tiger Claw"[IV], and 'Tiger Hiding in the Mountains'[V]. The technique used here is "The Fierce Tiger Lurking Under a Rock"[VI]. If the enemy approaches me, I

[I] **"Tiger Descends from the Mountain"** (下山虎, Mandarin: *XIA SHAN HU*, Cantonese: *HAA SAAN FU*) - This technique is described in detail by **Lam Sai Wing** in *Tiger and Crane,* **Fig. 63, [index, p. 226]**.

[II] **"Single Tiger Claw"** (單虎爪, Mandarin: *DAN HU ZHAO*, Cantonese: *DAAN FU ZAAU*), **[index, p. 224]**.

[III] **"Double Tiger Claw"** (雙虎爪, Mandarin: *SHUANG HU ZHAO*, Cantonese: *SEUNG FU ZAAU*), **[index, p. 217]**.

[IV] **"Black Tiger Claw"** (黑虎爪, Mandarin: *HEI HU ZHAO*, Cantonese: *HAAK FU ZAAU*) - a blow with a hand in the position *"Tiger Claw"* to the enemy's face with a subsequent grip and a squeeze (**Fig. 84**). This technique and its combat application are described in detail by **Lam Sai Wing** in *Tiger and Crane,* **Fig. 94, [index, p. 215]**. There is a method with a similar name *HEI HU SHOU – "Hand of Black Tiger"* among the called *"72 Secret Arts of Monks from the Shaolin Monastery"*. This method is intended to enhance the strength and hardness of fingers and nails, as well as the strength of a grip (Jin Jing Zhong. *Authentic Shaolin Heritage: Training Methods Of 72 Arts Of Shaolin*, Shaolin Kung Fu Online Library, 2008, **p. 207**).

[V] **"Tiger Hiding in the Mountains"** (隱山虎, Mandarin: *YIN SHAN HU*, Cantonese: *JAN SAAN FU*) **[index, p. 226]**.

[VI] **"Fierce Tiger Lurking Under a Rock"** (猛虎隱巖, Mandarin: *MENG HU YING YANG*, Cantonese: *MAANG FU JAN NGAAM*) – dodging an enemy attack by moving to a low *SEI PING MAA* stance with a deflecting block with the elbow and forearm (**Fig. 44**), **[index, p. 218]**.

immediately switch to the "Black Tiger Claw" technique and subdue him.

Commentaries: This technique is described in the commentaries to **Fig. 44**.

圖九十五

爪虎雙掙兜馬進

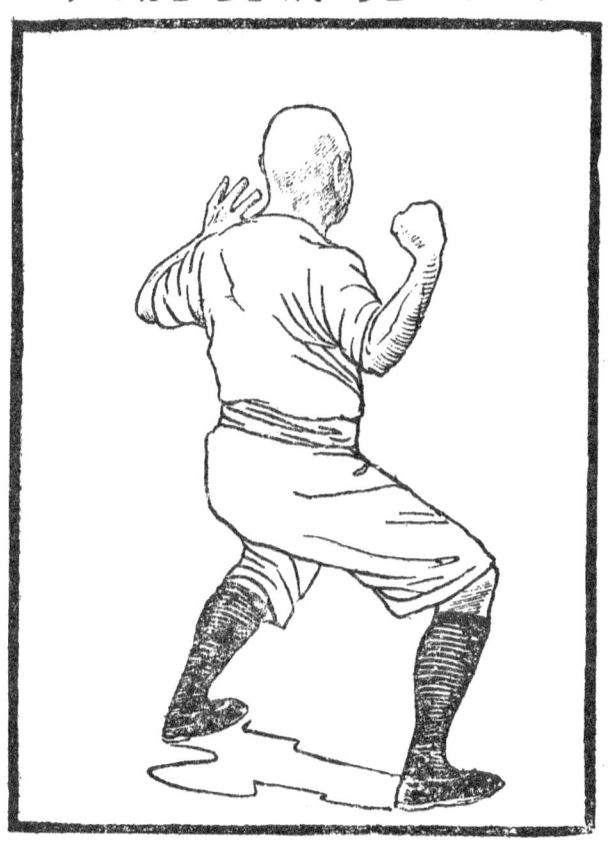

虎爪之法有開山虎下山虎單虎爪雙虎爪黑虎爪隱
山虎此虎爪乃猛虎隱巖之勢如敵人入我即轉黑
虎爪法服他

FIG. 59

六十　牛角一搥轉通天

NIU JIAO YI CHUI ZHUAN TONG TIAN (Mandarin)
NGAU GOK JAT CEOI JYUN TUNG TIN (Cantonese)

60. The Bull Strikes with Its Horn, Go On and Breach the Sky.

It is necessary to deliver the blow "The Bull Strikes with Its Horn"[I] to the enemy's head. "The Blow that Breaches the Sky"[II] is delivered to the enemy's chin. Manchu[III] men, moving forward three steps, attack me with three punches "The Bull Strikes with Its Horn". If he attacks me in this manner, I immediately lower myself to the stance "Four Levels Eight Parts Horse Stance"[IV] and use "Pulling Arrow Fist"[V]. I deliver a blow and win an easy victory.

[I] *"The Bull Strikes with Its Horn"* (牛角搥, Mandarin: *NIU JIAO CHUI*, Cantonese: *NGAU GOK CEOI*) – a circular punch delivered with the elbow bent (similar to a hook in boxing) **(Fig. 45), [index, p. 215]**.

[II] *"The Blow that Breaches the Sky"* (通天搥, Mandarin: *TONG TIAN CHUI*, Cantonese: *TUNG TIN CEOI*) – punch from down to up (similar to an uppercut in boxing) **[index, p. 215]**.

[III] The *Manchu* (滿洲) are an ethnic group originating from *Manchuria*, in northeastern *China*.

[IV] *"Stable Horse Riding Stance"* (四平八分馬, Mandarin: *SEI PING BA FEN MA*, Cantonese: *SEI PING BAAT FAN MAA*) – literally: *"Four Levels Eight Parts Horse Stance"* - lower *"Horse Stance"*, i.e., the feet are widespread, the center of gravity is situated low **(Fig. 10), [see index, p. 225]**.

[V] *"Pulling Arrow Fist"* (猛箭拳, Mandarin: *MENG JIAN QUAN*, Cantonese: *MANG JIN KYUN*), full name: *"Draw the Bow and Shoot the Arrow"* (猛弓射箭, Mandarin: *MENG GONG SHE JIAN*, Cantonese: *MANG GUNG SE JIN*) - see text and commentaries to Fig. 83, **[index, p. 223]**.

Commentaries: see commentaries to **Fig. 45**. Here, the author describes a possible counterattack, if the enemy tries to use a series of blows *"The Bull Strikes with Its Horn"* against you.

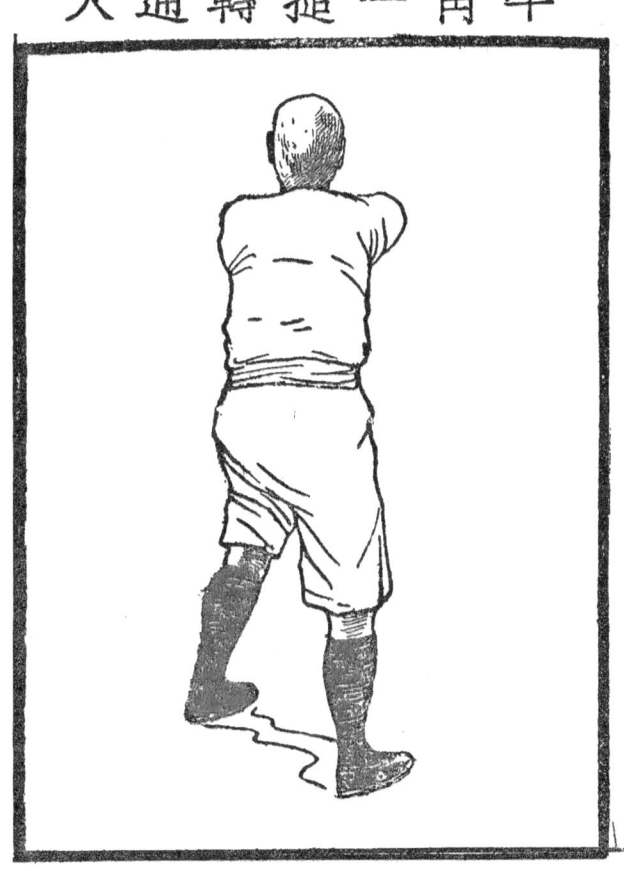

圖十六

牛角一挑轉通天

牛角挑須打敵人頭部通天挑須打他人下扒滿洲人。
牛角拳連環起脚一出三打之法若他來我即用八分
四平馬用搖箭拳破之無難

FIG. 60

六十一　坐馬單橋搥進步

ZUO MA DAN QIAO CHUI JIN BU (Mandarin)
JO MAA DAAN KIU CEOI ZEON BOU (Cantonese)

61. Sit in a Stance, Single Bridge, Move Forward One Step with a Blow.

In the moment when the enemy attacks me on the middle level and delivers a fist blow, I immediately turn my body and parry that blow with my "Bridge" (forearm)[I]. Without stopping, I immediately move forward to a strong position and hit the enemy with a punch. After putting a "Bridge" in front, it is necessary to advance to the firm position and deliver a crushing punch to the enemy's side, his heart, or his breast. If you do not move forward in your position when you strike, your blow will be lacking in power, and you will not be able to knock down your opponent.

Commentaries: A blow is parried with a forearm in the low **Horse Stance (SEI PING BAAT FAN MAA)**, your left side faces the enemy (**Fig. 86**). Then your left foot makes a half step forward, and you pass into the stance **The Bow and the Arrow (JI NG MAA)**. Your right fist should hit the target at the moment of turning your body. At the same time as the blow, the left hand is pulled up to your waist. Thus, the coordinated work of arms, body, and legs is achieved. In this case, the blow is strong enough to defeat the enemy. There should not be pauses between the block and the blow, one movement smoothly turns into another. **Fig. 61** shows the moment of striking with the right fist. The same blow is shown at another angles in **Fig. 70** and **Fig. 71**.

[I] A transversal block with a forearm, a hand in the position "a single finger," this posture is shown in **Fig. 86**.

六十一圖
坐馬單橋搪進步

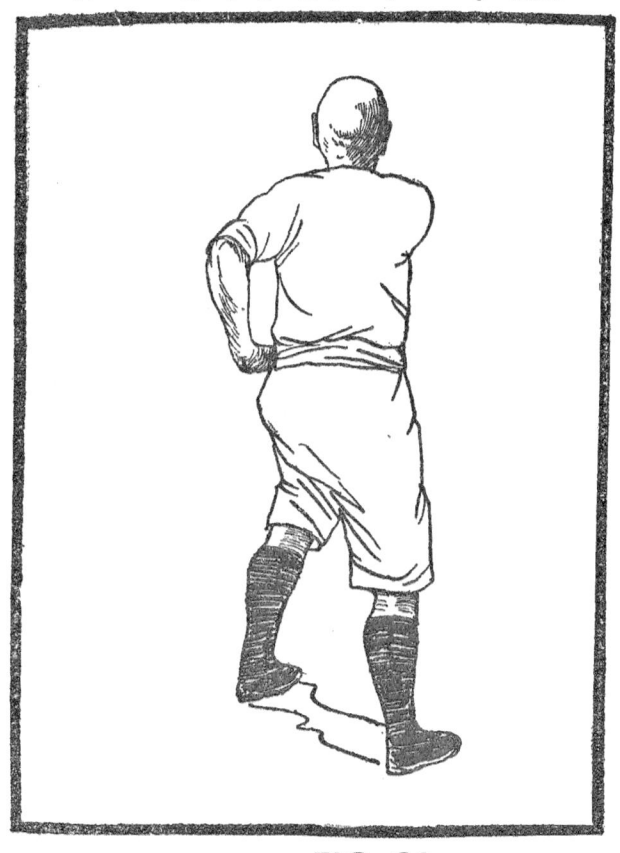

FIG. 61

此勢倘敵人中拳打來我即轉身對膊一橋連環進馬一拳打出一橋之後必要進馬冲拳方到敵者心胸若不進馬而發拳則不能傷他

六十二　拉馬一頂磟掙撇

LA MA YI DING LU ZHENG PIE (Mandarin)
LAAI MAA JAT DENG LUK ZAANG PIT (Cantonese)

62. Rein in the Horse, Elbow Like a Stone Pestle, Diagonal Downward Elbow.

This method is appropriate when I engage one enemy in front of me and another enemy appears behind and attacks me. I immediately "Rein in the Horse", turn back, and deliver a blow with my elbow's tip. This is the technique "Elbow Like a Stone Pestle."[I] The enemy presses on my elbow to eliminate my attack. Without interrupting the movement, I move on to the technique "Diagonal Downward Elbow"[II] and beat off the enemy. At this moment, the first enemy left behind me attacks me with a blow to my head. I quickly turn around in the MAA stance, parry his blow, and hit him with the "Hand of 1000 Characters".

Commentaries: From the previous position (**Fig. 61**), turn to the right to 90 degrees and take the *"Horse Stance"*. At the same time, deliver a straight blow with the tip of your right elbow to the enemy's breast or abdomen. If the enemy blocks your blow,

---

[I] *"Elbow Like a Stone Pestle"* (頂磟, Mandarin: **DING LU**, Cantonese: **DENG LUK**) - a straight strike with the tip of the elbow to the side, horizontally, at shoulder level (**Fig. 23**), [index, p. 217].

[II] *"Diagonal Downward Elbow"* (掙撇, Mandarin: **ZHENG PIE**, Cantonese: **ZAANG PIT**) - the striking elbow moves in a downward diagonal path to target areas like the opponent's forehead, eyebrow, or cheek. To perform the blow, you need to raise your elbow up and to the side, approximately at the level of the forehead, the hand is near the chin, and then slash it down at an angle, often incorporating body weight and rotation for power; the blow can be used to break an opponent's guard [index, p. 216].

take the right stance *JI NG MAA* (*"The Bow and the Arrow"*) and deliver a "***Diagonal Downward Elbow***" blow with your left elbow. Then, without changing your stance, deliver a side blow with your right elbow. This blow is shown in **Fig. 62**. If another enemy at this moment attacks you from behind with a blow aimed at your head, turn back on your left foot, step with your right foot, and take the ***SEI PING MAA*** (*"Horse Stance"*).

圖 二 十 六

撇 胂 碌 頂 一 馬 拉

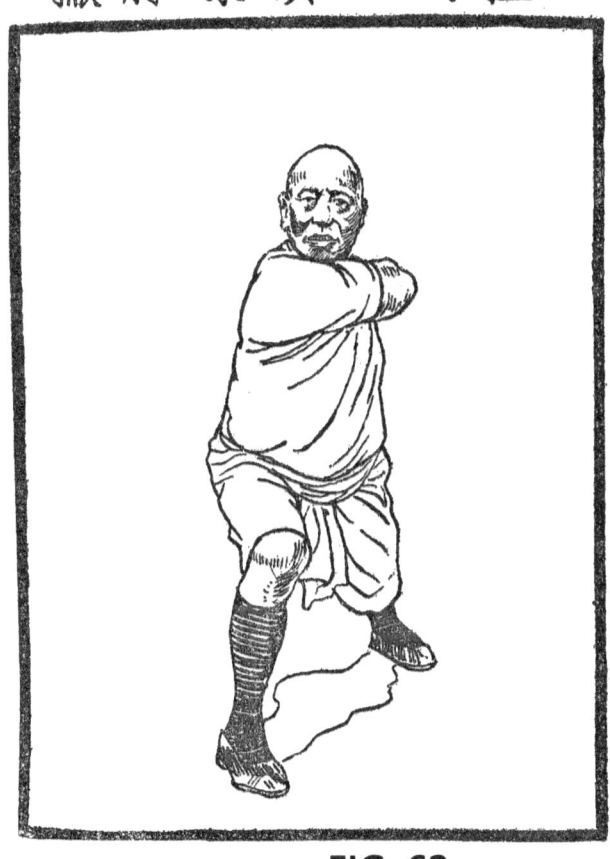

此勢即與前面交手若後面有敵至我即拉馬向後一
頂胂頂他敵人用迫胂消我連一扒一頂我用碌頂胂
消之再由後頭部打來我即縮馬轉身連環扣打上馬
千字攻之

FIG. 62

Simultaneously with the arrival in the stance, perform the technique ***"Hand of 1000 Characters "*** with your right arm. In this case, this technique can be used as a block or as a counterattack. The movement is performed with a wide swinging motion, from top to bottom, diagonally. The right arm is almost completely straightened at the elbow. In the final phase, the open left palm meets the right forearm near the left hip.

六十三　匝頭蝶掌莫延遲

HUI TOU DIE ZHANG MO YAN CHI (Mandarin)
WUI TAU DIP JEUNG MOK JIN CI (Cantonese)

63. Turn the Head and Perform the Butterfly Palms Without Delay.

If the opponent approaches from behind and intends to strike, I immediately twist my body and pull both hands towards me, turn my head, and turn around. I parry the enemy's strike with the "Butterfly Palms"[I] and strike back. To do this, I move forward and use the "Black Tiger Claw"[II] technique to restrain the opponent.

Commentaries: After performing the *"Hand of 1000 Hieroglyphs"* technique, turn to the opponent attacking you from behind and perform the *"Palms like Butterflies"* technique (**Fig. 63**). Then step forward with your right foot into the *JI NG MAA* (*"The Bow and the Arrow"*) stance and perform the *"Black Tiger Claw"* technique. This technique is

---

[I] *"Palms like Butterflies"* (蝶掌, Mandarin: *DIE ZHANG*, Cantonese: *DIP JEUNG*) - circular block with both palms in the frontal plane, followed by a simultaneous blow with open palms at two levels, the fingers of the upper palm are directed upwards, the fingers of the lower palm are directed downwards (**Figs. 52, 63, 66, 89**), **[see index, p. 223]**.

[II] *"Black Tiger Claw"* (黑虎爪, Mandarin: *HEI HU ZHAO*, Cantonese: *HAAK FU ZAAU*) - a blow with a hand in the position *"Tiger Claw"* to the enemy's face with a subsequent grip and a squeeze (**Fig. 84**) **[see index, p. 215]**.

described in the text and commentaries to **Fig. 84**. See also:
Lam Sai Wing. *Tiger and Crane*, **Fig. 94**.

圖 三 十 六
遲延莫掌蝶頭回

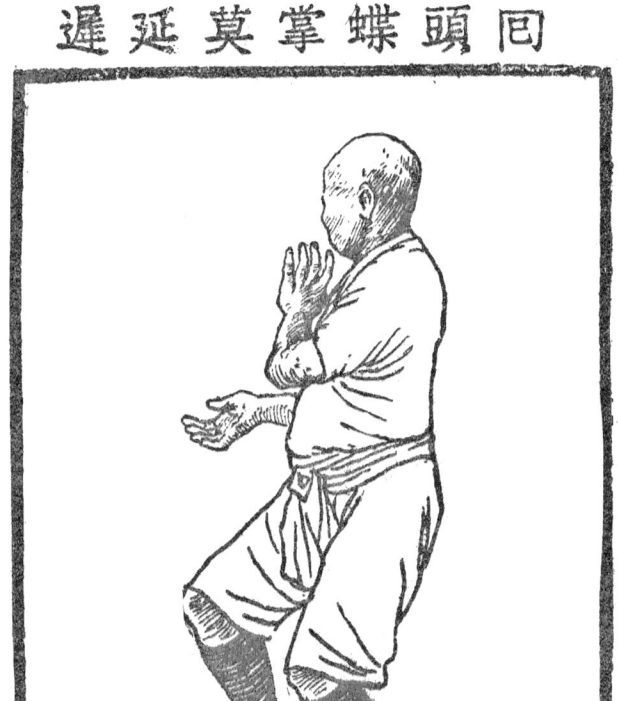

如敵人由後打來我即扭身轉後雙手一撒即回頭蝶
掌之法連消帶打再進馬用黑虎爪法迫他

FIG. 63

六十四　黑虎捶法連環打

HEI HU CHUI FA LIAN HUAN DA (Mandarin)
HAAK FU CEOI FAAT LIN WAAN DAA (Cantonese)

64. The Black Tiger Delivers a Blow and a Continuous Series of Blows.

To successfully use the Black Tiger Strike, you need to stay close to the enemy, you need to follow him as if "glued". Then step to the other side, facing the next enemy, block his strike with the "Arm Like a Wing"[1] and then, in one move, punch him in the shape of the character "Sun" (日) at a medium level.

Commentaries: After performing the "***Black Tiger Claw***" technique, turn 180 degrees to the left into the ***SEI PING MA*** *("Horse Stance")* and parry the enemy's strike with the left ***Arm Like a Wing***" (elbow bent at a right angle, forearm vertical, palm facing inward). Then, without changing the position of your feet and your left arm, assume the ***JI NG MAA*** (*"The Bow and the Arrow"*) stance and deliver a straight punch with your right vertical fist at mid-level (elbow slightly bent at the final phase of the strike).

---

[1] *Arm Like a Wing"* (膀手, Mandarin: *BANG SHOU*, Cantonese: *BONG SAU*), a forearm block, **[see index, p. 215]**.

圖四十六
打環連法搥虎黑

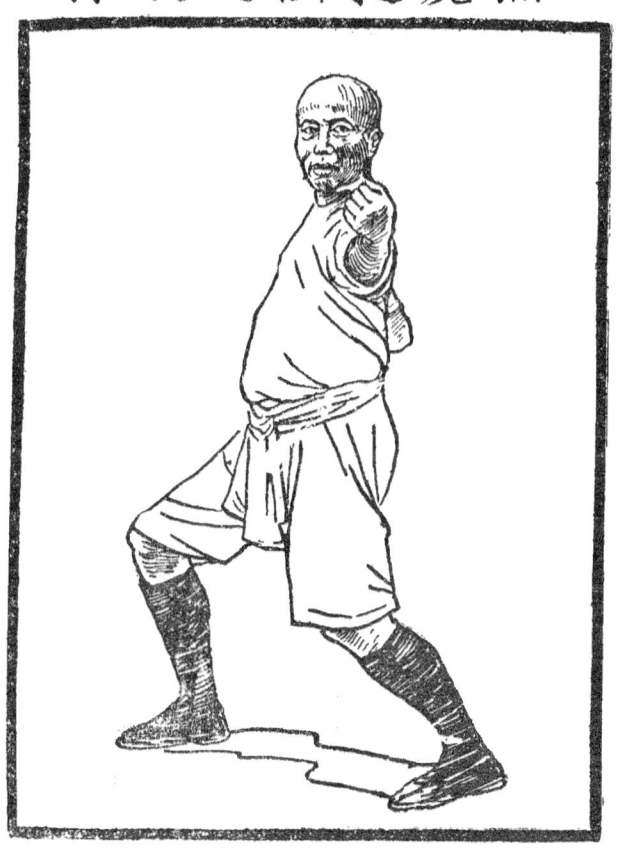

黑虎搥法須與敵人貼近身邊隨行由側面打他他用
膀手招我我連馬用日字拳打他腰部

FIG. 64

六十五　蝴蝶一掌麒麟步

HU DIE YI ZHANG QI LIN BU (Mandarin)
WU DIP JAT JEUNG KEI LEON BOU (Cantonese)

65. Palms Like Butterflies, the Unicorn Step[I].

If the enemy attacks me from behind with a blow at my waist, I immediately make a step forward with my right foot, pull my left foot towards my right foot, and perform a continuous series of "Butterfly Palms"[II] techniques to the left and right sides.

Commentaries: Take a step forward with your right foot from the left posture ***JI NG MAA*** (*'The Bow and the Arrow'*) and assume the stance shown in **Fig. 65**. At the same time, parry the enemy's attack at the middle level with the back of your right palm and your right forearm. Without stopping, turn on your right foot to 180 degrees clockwise. At the same time, your left foot rounds your right foot and returns to the previous place. Your hands in the position "claws" hold an initial position to deliver a blow with "palms like butterflies": the left hand is near your waist, the right hand is near your left shoulder. Thus, you find yourself facing the enemy who attacked you behind your back. Then make a step forward with your right foot into the stance ***JI NG MAA*** (*'The Bow and the Arrow'*) and deliver a double blow with the ***"Palms like Butterflies"***, this

---

[I] ***"Unicorn Step"*** (麒麟步, Mandarin: ***QI LIN BU***, Cantonese: ***KEI LEON BOU***) - a specific footwork technique that allows you to turn in any direction at the desired angle in two movements (steps). First, step with the back foot, placing it in front of the front foot, close to it, with knees close together, and shift the body weight forward. Then, pivot on the front foot to the desired angle and step forward with the back foot. In this form, this step is used when performing the ***"Butterfly Palms"*** technique to perform a 180-degree turn (two steps, one after the other). **Figs. 95, 96, [see index, p. 227].**

[II] ***"Palms like Butterflies"*** (蝶掌, Mandarin: ***DIE ZHANG***, Cantonese: ***DIP JEUNG***) - **[see index, p. 223].**

time your right palm is in the upper position and the left one is in the lower position. All the movements should be done quickly and smoothly, without pauses.

蝴蝶一掌麒麟步

此勢如敵人用拳打我腰部我即將右腳退前歸左蝶掌一搨連環一掌即左右蝶掌之法

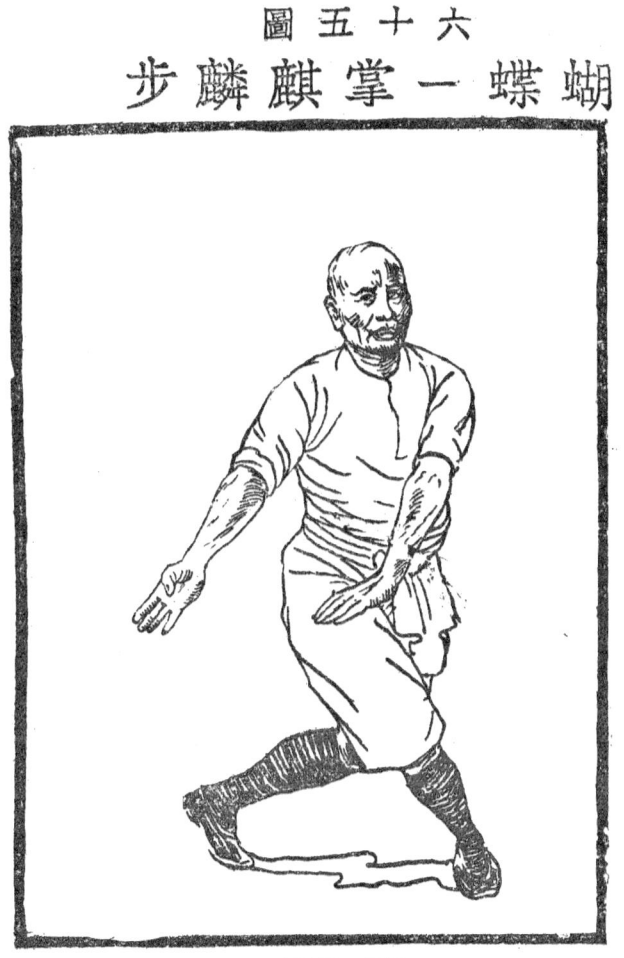

FIG. 65

六十六 連環蝶掌步麒麟

LIAN HUAN DIE ZHANG BU QI LIN (Mandarin)
LIN WAAN DIP JEUNG BOU KEI LEON (Cantonese)

66. Continuous Series of Palms Like Butterflies in the Unicorn Movement.

If an enemy tries to kick me from behind, I use the "Unicorn Step," parry his attack, and immediately strike him with the "Palms like Butterflies." This technique does not require much strength: I deflect the strike with "Butterfly Palms," immediately follow up with "Divide and Penetrate with Hands,"[I] and strike the enemy.

Commentaries: Now the ***"Palms like Butterflies"*** technique (and the "***Unicorn Step***") are performed in the opposite direction (at a 45-degree angle to the centerline). This results in a left-handed ***JI NG MAA*** (*"Bow and Arrow"*) stance, with your left palm in the upper position, and your right one in the lower position.

[I] *"Turn and Divide, Penetrate with Hands"* (轉分漏手, Mandarin: ***ZHUAN FEN LOU SHOU***, Cantonese: ***JYUN FAN LAU SAU***) - see commentaries on page 44, **[see index, p. 226]**.

圖 六十

連環蝶掌步麒麟

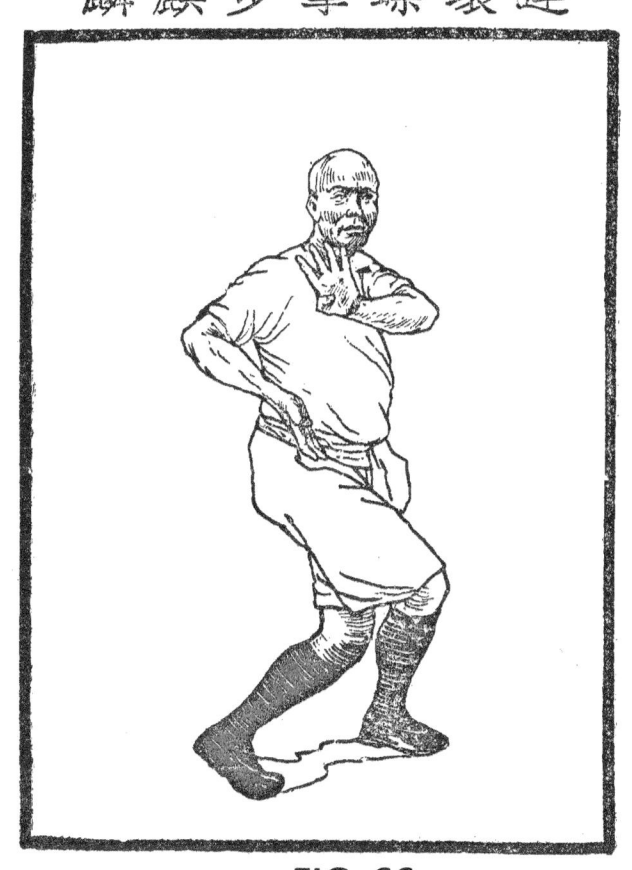

倘敵人打我後腿我用麒麟步手用蝴蝶掌連環打出
他人力大不招架我即變蝶掌分漏手打他

FIG. 66

六十七　右抽一拳連打出

YOU CHOU YI QUAN LIAN DA CHU (Mandarin)
JAU CAU JAT KYUN LIN DAA CHEUT (Cantonese)

67. Pull Out the Right Fist, Simultaneously Moving Forward with a Punch.

This is a technique for simultaneously blocking and striking. It does not matter which technique the enemy uses against me; all the same, I use the method "One Block, One Strike." When I use this kind of blow, I do as if I were squeezing a wooden billet with my elbows and strike right and left. I advance, turn, block, and deliver blows.

Commentaries: Step your right foot forward and to the right, at a 45-degree angle to the center line, and assume a right-handed **JI NG MAA** (*"Bow and Arrow"*) stance. At the same time, block the enemy's blow aimed at your head or breast with a motion of your right forearm from inside to outside and deliver a straight blow with your left fist (**Fig. 67**). Make sure to keep your right elbow down and pointed downward to protect your right chest from a possible counterattack from your opponent.

圖七十六
出打連拳一抽右

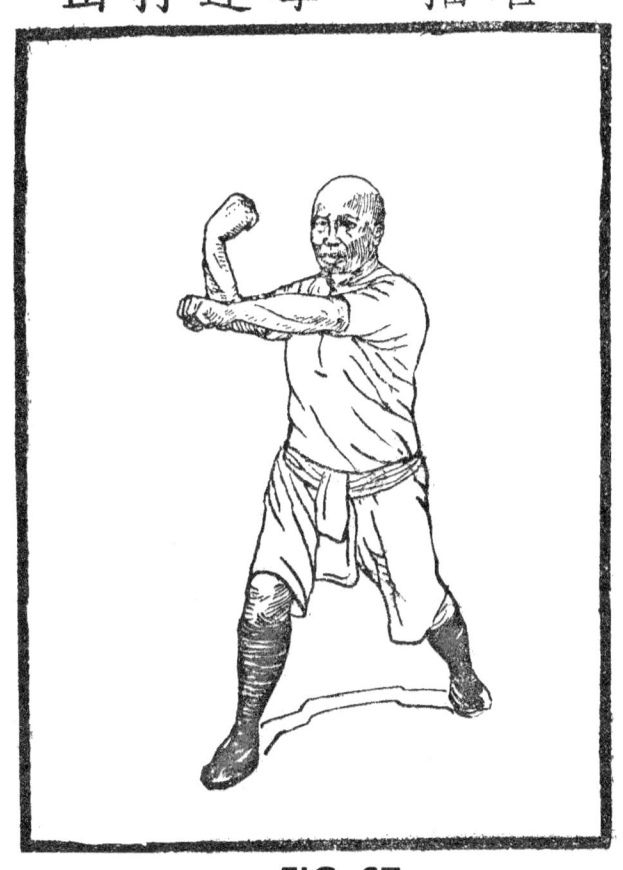

一抽一拳之法無論何法我用一抽一搥招之此拳連
環夾木搥左右進步連轉扣打拳法

FIG. 67

六十八　左右連環一樣同

ZUO YOU LIAN HUAN YI YANG TONG (Mandarin)
JO JAU LIN WAAN JAT JOENG TUNG (Cantonese)

68. Left and Right, Continuously and Sequentially, Perform the Same Technique.

This is a continuous chain of movements: first, the right foot steps forward into a JI NG MAA ("Bow and Arrow") stance, the right hand is pulled in, and the left hand punches. Then, without stopping, in a continuous series of movements, the left foot steps forward and to the left, the left hand is pulled in, and the right hand punches. Thus, the technique is performed in a continuous series to the left and right. This technique is called "Squeeze a Wooden Billet and Punch."[I]

Commentaries: Here, the author describes the continuous execution of the *"Squeeze a Wooden Billet and Punch"* technique, first to the right (**Fig. 67**) and then to the left (**Fig. 68**), at a 45-degree angle to the front.

After performing the technique to the right (**Fig. 67**), lower your left elbow to the left side of your breast and pull the left fist to yourself. At the same time, make a step with your left foot to the left and forward, and deliver a straight blow with your right fist. While you are performing the series of two blows, your elbows should protect your breast at all times; they should not be set aside. At the final stage of the strike, your

---

[I] *"Squeeze a Wooden Billet and Punch"* (夾木拳, Mandarin: *JIA MU QUAN*, Cantonese: *GAAP MUK KYUN*) - a block with the front arm, and simultaneously punch with the rear arm. At the final stage of the strike, your elbows should be fairly close together, as if you're squeezing a wooden billet between your elbows, preventing it from falling **[index, p. 225]**.

elbows should be fairly close together, as if you're squeezing a wooden billet between your elbows, preventing it from falling.

第六十八圖

左右連環一樣同

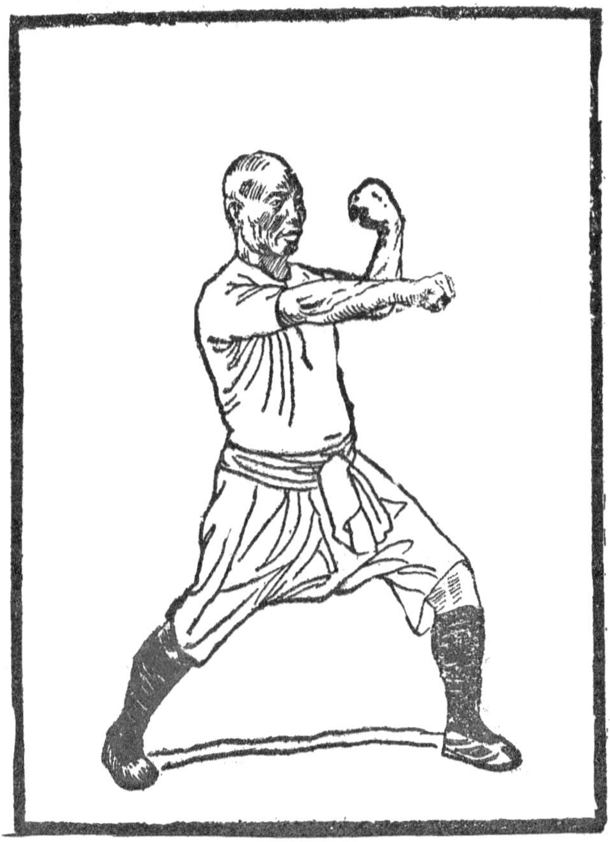

此法用右脚上子午馬右手一抽左手一拳連環招打
左手一抽右手一拳打歸左即是連環夾木拳之法

FIG. 68

六十九　轉身單掛搥中出

ZHUAN SHEN DAN GUA CHUI ZHONG CHU (Mandarin)
JYUN SAN DAAN GWA CEOI JUNG CHEUT (Cantonese)

69. Turn Around, Single Overhanging Fist, Go On With the Punch Toward the Center.

A high stance is not appropriate here. Turn your body, deliver the "Overhanging Fist"[I] blow, and immediately follow it up with a straight punch to the center. Turn back, pull your fist toward you after delivering the "Overhanging Fist" blow, and immediately follow it up with a straight punch to the center. Change your stance again and, in a single sequence of strikes, deliver the "Overhanging Blow" and immediately deliver a straight punch to the center. Thus, the technique is performed in three directions, the pattern of movements similar to the character "品".

Commentaries: From the left-handed stance of *"Squeeze a Wooden Billet and Punch"* (**Fig. 68**), turn right clockwise 135 degrees to the right-handed *JI NG MAA* (*"Bow and Arrow"*) stance. At the same time, deliver the blow *GUA* (*"Overhanging Fist"*) with the back of the right fist and the straight punch *CHUI* at the middle level with the left fist. The *GUA* is delivered immediately after the turn in motion, when you pass into the right-handed stance *JI NG MAA*, and the left fist blow is delivered at the moment of putting your right foot on the ground. Then make a turn on your right foot to 180 degrees anti-clockwise, pass into the left stance *JI NG MAA*, and do the technique to the other side: the *GUA* with your left fist, and the straight punch *CHUI* with the right one. This

---

I *"Overhanging Fist"* (掛拳, Mandarin: *GUA QUAN*, Cantonese: *GWA KYUN*) - blow (or a block) with the back side of the fist and (or) the outer side of the forearm delivered from up to down. The fist moves from the shoulder level to the waist, making a semi-circle in the vertical plane (**Fig. 69**) **[index, p. 222]**.

position is shown in **Fig. 70**. Then step your right foot to the right and turn 90 degrees clockwise (you should be standing with your back to the initial point from which you started to execute *TAO*) and perform the technique again in a right-handed stance. That position is illustrated in **Fig. 71**. Thus, the trajectory of your movements is similar to the character "**品**": you perform the technique three times - to the right, then to the left, and then forward.

六十九圖

轉身單掛搥中出

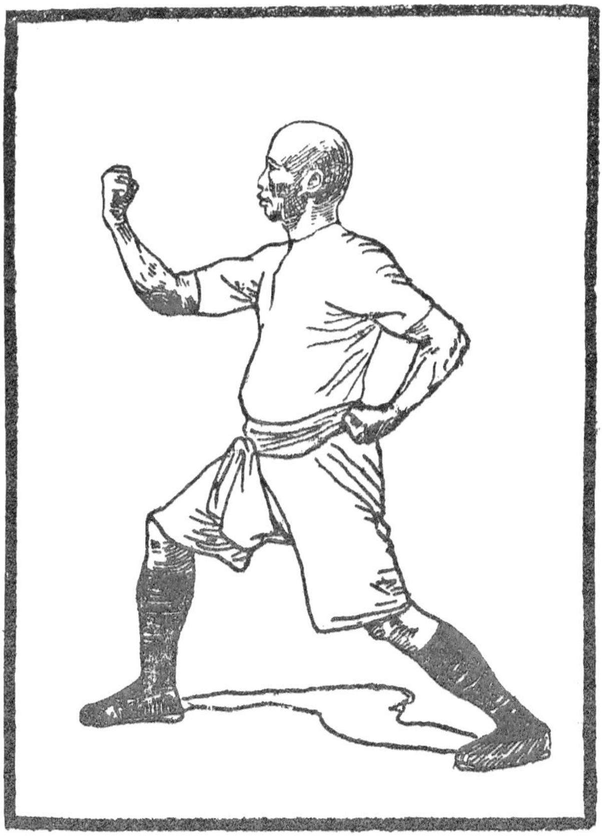

此勢不用上馬轉身掛打一拳連環一中拳擰身拉後
掛打了拳連環一中拳連上馬掛打打正又連環掛打
中拳卽品字樣一般

FIG. 69

七十　拉馬轉身掛打搥

LA MA ZHUAN SHEN GUA DA CHUI (Mandarin)
LAAI MAA JYUN SAN GWA DAA CEOI (Cantonese)

70. Take the Horse by the Reins, Turn Around, Overhanging Blow with the Punch.

This "Overhanging Blow and Punch"[I] technique was passed down to us as a legacy of the Shaolin Temple. One "Overhanging Fist" blow and one Punch – this technique is performed three times in a row, in a continuous series, one after the other. The orthodox Shaolin version of the technique involves performing the series in a straight line. Thanks to Wong Fei Hung's refinement, movements to the left, right, and forward were added to the technique. Thus, the movement pattern resembles the character "品".

Commentaries: The series of three consecutive *"Overhanging Blow and Punch"* continues: **Fig. 70** shows the second strike in the series (to the left of the center line with the right fist).

See commentaries to **Fig. 69**.

[I] *"Overhanging Blow and Punch"* (掛打搥, Mandarin: *GUA DA CHUI*, Cantonese: *GWA DAA CEOI*) - the technique involves two blows performed one after the other: the *GWA* ("*Overhanging* Fist", see index p. 222) with the front hand, followed by a *CEOI* (straight punch) with the back hand **[index, p. 221]**.

拉馬轉身掛打搥

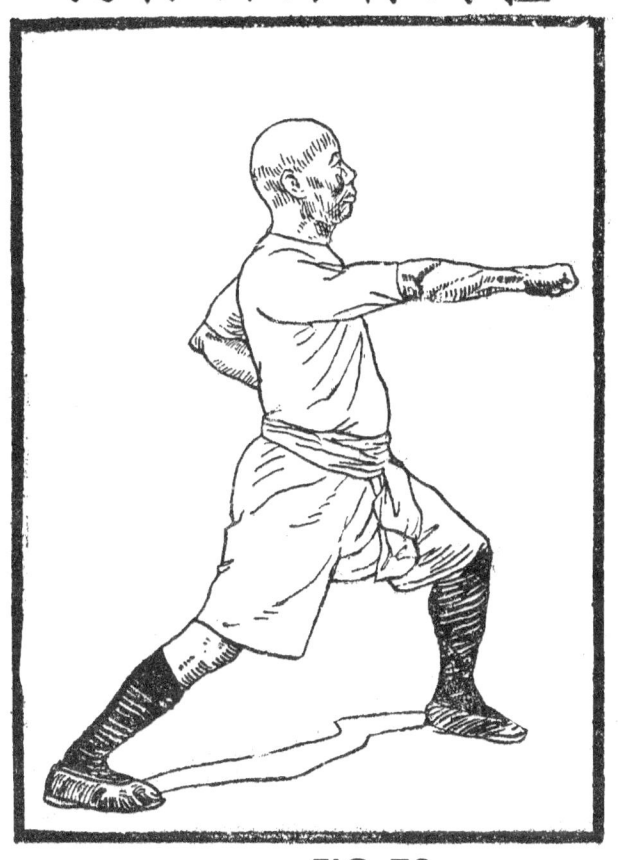

FIG. 70

此掛打搥法由少林寺傳授之法一掛一拳連轉三拳
是少林之正宗因黃飛鴻改造左右前後掛打拳轉作
品字樣掛打拳法

七十一　向前掛打連環落

XIANG QIAN GUA DA LIAN HUAN LUO (Mandarin)
HOENG CIN GWA DAA LIN WAAN LOK (Cantonese)

71. Turn Forward, Overhanging Blow, Complete the Sequence.

When performing the technique "Overhanging Blow and Punch", you must resolutely advance forward step by step, attacking without retreating or pausing. The "Overhanging Blow" and Straight Punch follow one another in a continuous sequence. Press forward without hesitation. Only in this way can this technique be applied successfully.

Commentaries: Fig. 71 shows the third (final in this series) *"Overhanging Blow and Punch"*. It is delivered along the centerline. When you use the method ***GWA DAA CEOI*** ("***Overhanging Blow and Punch***") in a fight, it is necessary to "enter" the enemy quickly and resolutely, to disarrange his defense with the blow ***GUA*** and to deliver a straight decisive punch to his breast or to his stomach.

See commentaries to **Fig. 69**.

向前掛打連環落
圖 一 十 七

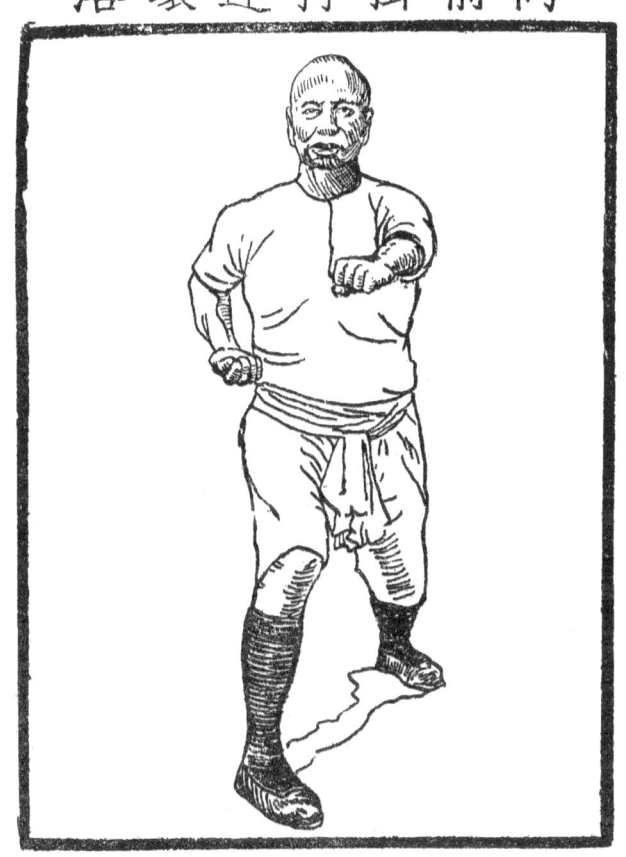

逢掛打拳步步進攻不可退後或停留一掛一拳連環進馬切莫停遲此法可用。

FIG. 71

七十二　後脚一拉千字手

HOU JIAO YI LA QIAN ZI SHOU (Mandarin)
HAU GEUK JAT LAAI CIN ZI SAU (Cantonese)

72. Pull Up Your Back Foot, Hand of 1000 Characters.

If the opponent attacks me from behind, I immediately turn back and apply the Hand of 1000 Characters[I] technique. My arm moves diagonally from the side of my body, my body slightly tilted. Then, without pause, I deliver a straight punch.

Commentaries: From a right-side stance *JI NG MAA* (*"Bow and Arrow"*), move your left foot slightly to the left and at the same time turn your torso 90 degrees counterclockwise. Take the *SEI PING MA* (*"Horse Stance"*) and block an enemy's blow from behind at the middle level with your left arm (**Fig. 72**). Then, without stopping, make a short step forward with your left foot, take the left-handed stance *JI NG MAA*, and deliver a straight fist blow to the enemy's breast or his stomach.

[I] *"The Hand of 1000 Characters"* (千字手, Mandarin: **QIAN ZI SHOU**, Cantonese: **CIN JI SAU**) - a wide range of blows and blocking with the arm (forearm), both from the inside out and the outside in, at different angles to the line of attack. The variations of this technique are shown in **Figs. 29, 35, 38, 42 [see index, p. 219]**. See also: *Lam Sai Wing, "Tiger and Crane"*.

七十二圖
後脚一拉千字手

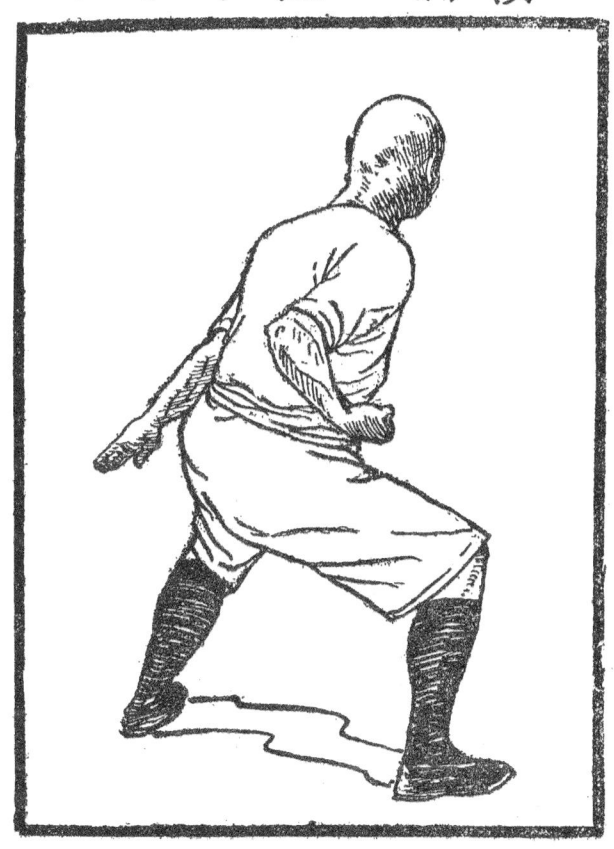

此勢如敵人由後打我即將後馬一拉用千字擸手
擸之此千字手須身側馬偏連環一拳打出

FIG. 72

七十三　進馬一搥頂睜出

JIN MA YI CHUI DING ZHENG CHU (Mandarin)
JEON MAA JAT CEOI DENG ZAANG CHEUT (Cantonese)

73. Move Forward in the Stance MAA, Strike With the Tip of the Elbow Outward.

The enemy lunges at me, brimming with energy and fury. I immediately advance in the stance MAA and strike him with the tip of my elbow. Then, without stopping or breaking movement, I hit him in the groin and immediately follow with an "Overhanging Blow" to the head. This is the "Overhanging Fist"[1] technique.

Commentaries: From the previous position, step forward with your right foot, turn to 90 degrees anticlockwise, and take the **SEI PING MA** (*"Horse Stance"*). At the same time as you come into a stance, deliver a straight blow with your right elbow tip on the middle level, then immediately strike with your right palm on the enemy's groin. In this moment, the hand is in the position *"Tiger Claw"*, the body is slightly tilted to the front and to the right. Without lingering in this position, deliver the ***"Overhanging Blow"*** to his face with your right fist. All three blows should be delivered quickly and precisely, without any pause.

---

[1] *"Overhanging Fist"* (掛拳, Mandarin: *GUA QUAN*, Cantonese: *GWA KYUN*) - blow (or a block) with the back side of the fist and (or) the outer side of the forearm delivered from up to down. The fist moves from the shoulder level to the waist, making a semi-circle in the vertical plane (Fig. 69) **[index, p. 222]**.

七十三圖

進馬一搥頂膌出

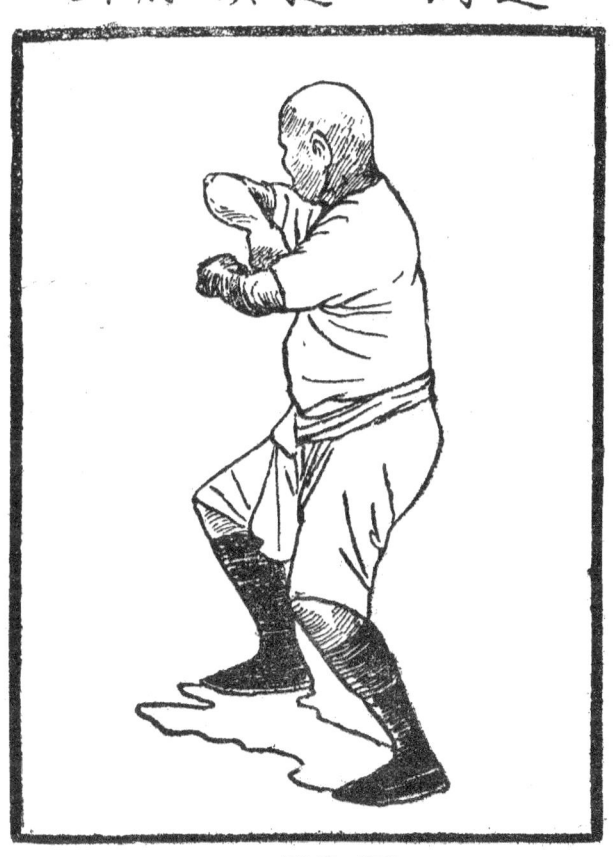

敵人來勢太猛我即用上馬一頂膌連環漏手打他陰部連環一掛打他頭部此法即單掛拳之法。

FIG. 73

七十四　分漏單掛轉金龍

FEN LOU DAN GUA ZHUAN JIN LONG (Mandarin)
FAN LAU DAAN GWA JYUN GAM LUNG (Cantonese)

74. Divide and Penetrate, Single Overhanging Fist, Transform Into the Golden Dragon.

Step back with your right foot, place it behind your left foot, and assume a SEI PING[I] stance. Whether the enemy attacks from above, in the middle, or below, you need not fear. By repeatedly using the "Hand of the Golden Dragon"[II] technique, you avoid numerous blows. Then pass to the stance JI NG[III] again and deliver a blow with your palm.

Commentaries: Step back with your right foot, turning your torso 90 degrees to the right, and assume a **SEI PING MAA** (*"Horse Stance"*). During this movement, lower your hands with open palms, then raise them through the sides to the head level. After that, cross your forearms in front of your breast with the centers of your palms facing your face. Then, without stopping the movement, push on the sides with your palms **(Fig. 74)**. Then, turn left 90 degrees, into a left-handed stance **JI NG MAA** (*"Bow and Arrow"*), and strike with your right palm.

[I] *"Horse Riding Stance"* (四平馬, Mandarin: *SEI PING MA*, Cantonese: *SEI PING MAA*) – literally: *"Four Levels Horse Stance"*, also known as the *"Horse Stance"* (馬步, *MA BU*), **[see index, p. 220]**.

[II] *"Hand of the Golden Dragon"* (金龍手, Mandarin: *JIN LONG SHOU*, Cantonese: *GAM LUNG SAU*) – a complex deflecting block technique that allows you to parry almost any enemy attack on all three levels (upper, middle and lower) **[index, p. 219]**.

[III] *JI NG MAA* (子午馬, Mandarin: *ZI WU MA*, Cantonese: *JI NG MAA*) - known in the modern *WUSHU* as the *"Bow and Arrow"* stance **[see index, p. 220]**.

七十四圖

分漏單掛轉金龍

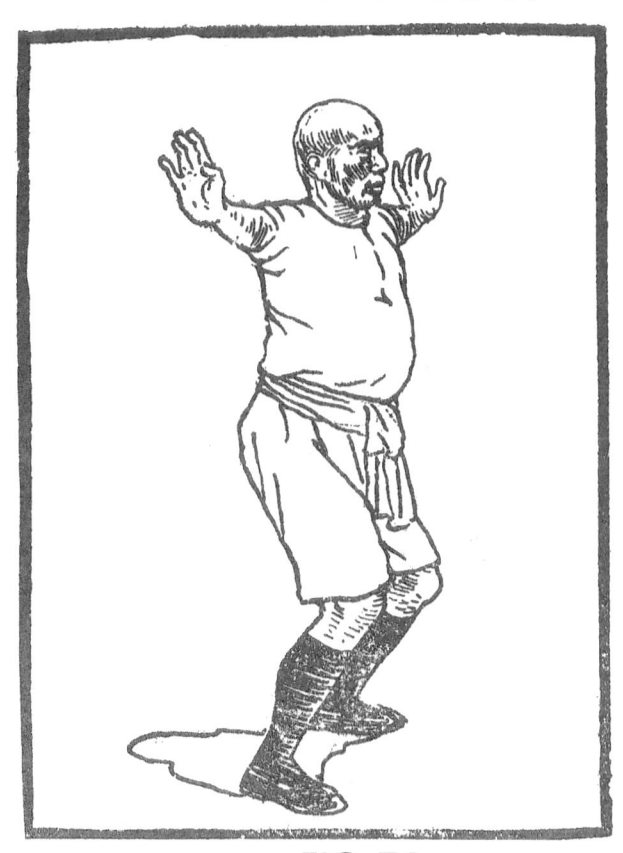

FIG. 74

退右脚落左四平無論敵人由上中下部打來我不用
驚心連轉金龍手法可保無虞再轉子午一掌打出

七十五　子午一掌虎尾脚

ZI WU YI ZHANG HU WEI JIAO (Mandarin)
JI NG JAT JEUNG FU MEI GEUK (Cantonese)

75. Palm Strike in JI NG Stance, The Tiger Tail Kick.

I strike with my palm in the JI NG stance, but the enemy grabs my wrist. I immediately pull my palm toward me, free myself, and grab him by the crook of his elbow. I execute the "Phoenix Eye"[I] strike and at once scratch at him with my claws. Without breaking movement, I lift my right foot and deliver a "Tiger Tail Kick"[II] at the waist level.

Commentaries: From the posture shown in **Fig. 74** your left foot makes one step forward and you take left-handed stance *JI NG MAA* (*"Bow and Arrow"*). Simultaneously you deliver a straight blow at the middle level with your right palm. If an opponent grabs your wrist, make a fist with your right hand and sharply and forcefully pull it toward your chest, simultaneously rotating your wrist. After releasing the grip, immediately grab the opponent's elbow with your right hand and, with your left hand in the *"Phoenix Eye"* position, strike their face. Then, without stopping the movement, the left and right hands in the *"Claws"* position move up and to the right and deliver a "scratching" blow to the opponent's face, moving down and to the left obliquely. Immediately after that, raise your right foot

––––––––––––––––––––––

[I] *"Phoenix Eye Fist"* (鳳眼拳, Mandarin: *FENG YAN QUAN*, Cantonese: *FUNG NGAAN KYUN*) – a technique focuses the power into a single point, specifically the second joint of the curled index finger, for striking vulnerable areas like the eye, temple, throat, solar plexus, etc. **[index, p. 223]**.

[II] *"The Tiger Tail Kick"* (虎尾脚, Mandarin: *HU WEI JIAO*, Cantonese: *FU MEI GEUK*) – a side kick, powerful, linear strike delivered with the heel or the entire outside edge of the foot; usually used to hit targets like the opponent's shins, knees, groin, or rib cage **(Fig. 75)**, . **[index, p. 226]**.

and deliver a ***"Tiger Tail Kick"*** with your heel at the level of the enemy's waist as shown in **Fig. 75**.

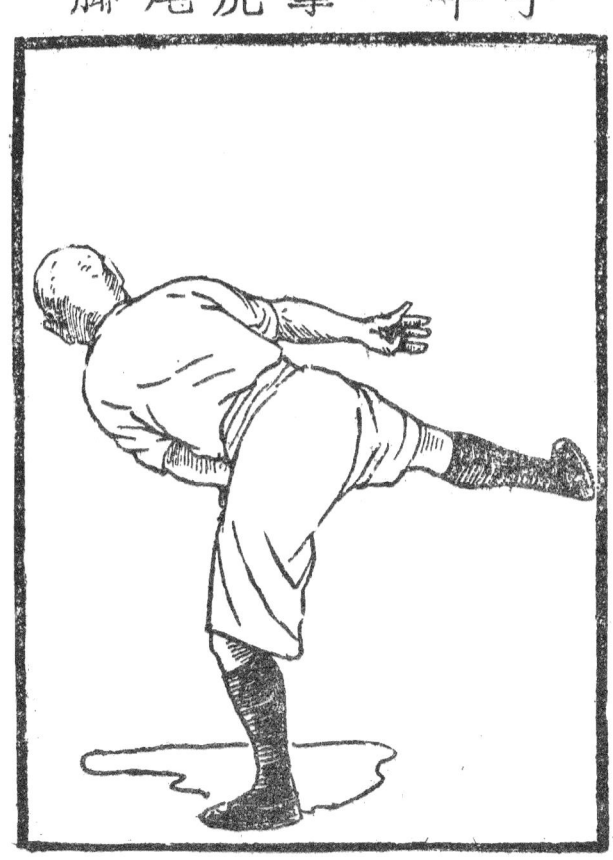

圖五十七
脚尾虎掌一午子

子午一掌逢敵人將我掌搭之我即用扒脖一揸用鳳
眼爪爪他連環起虎尾脚打他腰部。

FIG. 75

七十六 轉身蛇形又搶珠

ZHUAN SHEN SHE XING YOU QIANG ZHU (Mandarin)
JYUN SAN SE JING JAU COENG ZYU (Cantonese)

76. Turn Around, Snake Shape, Snatching the Pearls.

Turn around and use the method "Two Dragons Snatching Pearls"[I]. "Two Dragons Snatching Pearls" is a "Snake-Shaped Hand Technique"[II]. When using the "Snake-Shaped Hand Technique", the fingertips deliver piercing strikes into the opponent's body. Hakka[III] people are adept at using this technique, making it very difficult to counter.

Commentaries: After a kick (**Fig. 75**), pull your right foot toward your left knee, simultaneously pivoting 180 degrees counterclockwise on your left foot, and return your right foot to the same position it was in before the kick. Shift your weight to your right leg and bend it at the knee, keeping your left foot in place. Extend your left arm downward, parrying the opponent's low kick with an open palm. Without pausing in this position, shift your body weight forward and move into a

---

I *"Two Dragons Snatching Pearls"* (二龍搶珠, Mandarin: *ER LONG QIANG ZHU*, Cantonese: *JI LUNG COENG ZYU*) – a thrust into the enemy's eyes with the tips of the index and middle fingers, the remaining fingers pressed to the center of the palm (the character 珠, in addition to representing a pearl, also signifies the pupil of the eye), (**Fig. 76**), **[index, p. 227]**.

II *"Snake-Shaped Hand Technique"* (蛇形手法, Mandarin: *SHE XING SHOU FA*, Cantonese: *SE JING SAU FAAT*) – various fingertip strikes to vulnerable points on the enemy's body: the eyes, temples, throat, solar plexus, etc., **[index, p. 224]**.

III *"Hakka"* (客家, Mandarin: *KEJIA*, Cantonese: *HAAKGAA*) – a subgroup of the Han Chinese people known for their distinct culture, language, and history of migration. The term "Hakka" literally means "guest families," reflecting their history as migrants who moved in waves from northern China to southern China due to war, famine, and political unrest.

left-handed **JI NG MAA** (*"Bow and Arrow"*) stance, delivering a **"Snake-Shaped Hand"** strike to the opponent's eyes or throat. Depending on the target, the strike can be delivered with the tips of the index and middle fingers or the index and thumb.

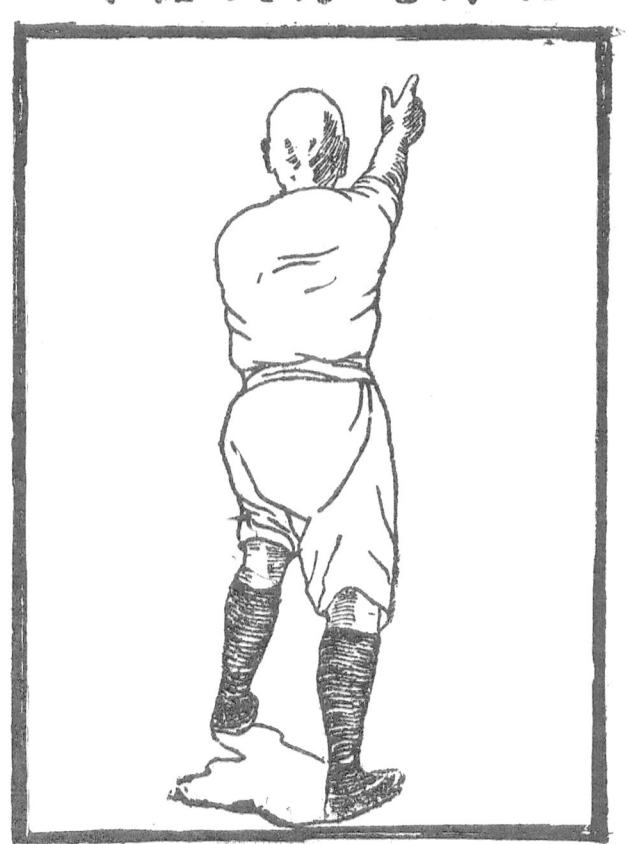

圖 六 十 七
珠 搶 又 形 蛇 身 轉

興身二龍搶珠即扰形三法逢蛇形手法用眼賀筆事
之勢客家人擅用此勢甚難招架

FIG. 76

七十七　飯匙頭起蛇擺尾

FAN SHI TOU QI SHE BAI WEI (Mandarin)
FAAN CI TAU HEI SE BAAI MEI (Cantonese)

77. Rice Spoon, Snake Raises Its Head, and Whipping Tail.

When performing the "Snake-Shaped Hand Technique", the palm is flat and the fingers are straight. The hand is quickly thrust forward and delivers a piercing strike with the fingertips — this is the BIAO CHUAN[I]. If the opponent presses against my (the striking) hand with a covering motion and attempts to control me, I immediately, without stopping, deliver piercing strikes BIAO CHUAN: from the left at an upward level, and from the right, with a downward motion from top to bottom, attacking him. If the opponent lifts his foot and intends to kick, I immediately apply the "Black Dragon Whipping Its Tail"[II] technique and successfully counter him.

Commentaries: After performing the previous technique (**Fig. 76**), clench your right hand into a fist and move it backward at the temple level; the wrist joint is bent at a right angle, and the forearm is vertical. That is the position *"**Rice Spoon**"[III]* (**Fig. 77**). If the enemy delivers you a blow at your head with his left arm, you deflect his blow aside with your right forearm, then, without stopping, immediately deliver a quick

---

[I] *"Do a Mark with a Piercing Hand"* (標串掌, Mandarin: *BIAO CHUAN ZHANG*, Cantonese: *BIU CYUN JEUNG*) - a thrust blow with the ends of fingers of an open palm [see index, p. 217].

[II] *"Black Dragon Whipping Its Tail"* (烏龍擺尾, Mandarin: *WU LONG BAI WEI*, Cantonese: *WU LUNG BAAI MEI*) – sweeping block at mid-level with both forearms in the *Unicorn Step* position (see commentaries to **Fig. 78**). See also: Lam Sai Wing, *Tiger and Crane*, **Fig. 79**, [index, p. 215].

[III] Chinese spoons differ in shape from Western spoons; they resemble small ladles.

stabbing blow ***BIAO CHUAN*** to the enemy's face with your fingertips (the right hand transforms from the position "fist" into the position "palm"). After the strike, the right arm immediately returns to the initial position: the wrist is bent, the forearm is vertical, and the palm is near the right temple.

圖七十七

尾擺蛇起頭匙飯

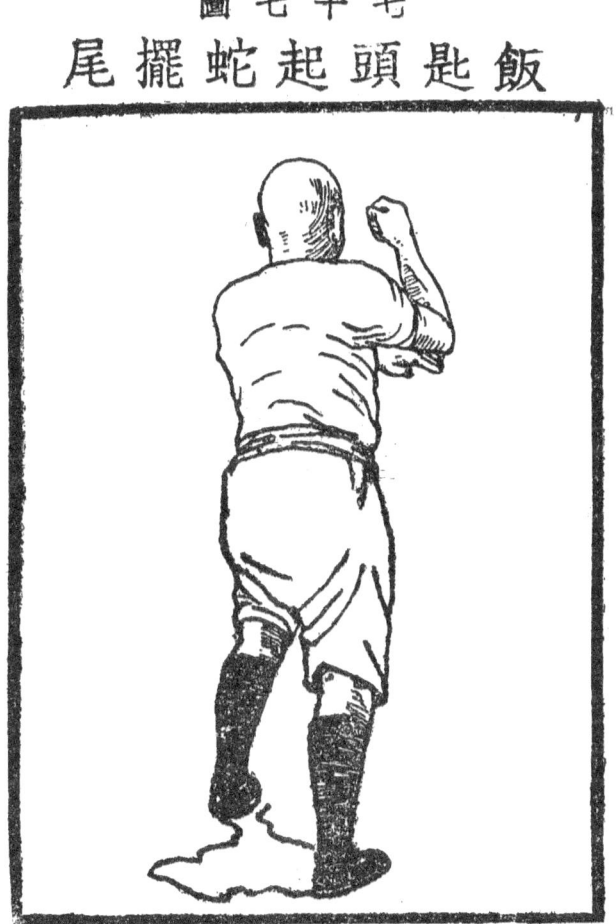

蛇形手法掌平指直一抽一標串敵人用刁手伏我我
即用連環標串左上右落之法攻之他起脚踢來我即
用烏龍擺尾之法招之

FIG. 77

That is the posture ***"Snake Raises Its Head"***. Your left palm, at waist level, protects the groin and abdomen from a possible attack with a foot or knee. Then proceed to the ***"Black Dragon Whipping Its Tail"*** technique (see commentaries for **Fig. 78**).

七十八　轉身一跳碌鼓搥

ZHUAN SHEN YI TIAO LU GU CHUI (Mandarin)
JYUN SAN JAT TIU LUK GU CEOI (Cantonese)

78. Turn Around, Jump, Beat the Drum With a Stone Pestle.

If in this situation the opponent attempts to attack me with a kick, I immediately retreat into a defensive stance, twist my body at the waist, and deliver a double-fisted downward GWA[I] blow with both fists, deflecting the enemy's kick—this is the "Black Dragon Whipping Its Tail" technique. Then, without stopping, I turn around and deliver successive GWA and PAAU[II] blows—this is the "Beat the Drum with a Stone Pestle"[III] technique.

Commentaries: From the left stance *JI NG MAA* (*"Bow and Arrow"*, **Fig. 77**), step forward with your right foot into position *"Unicorn Step"* (**Fig. 66**). Simultaneously twisting at the waist to the right, clench your hands into fists, and blocking the opponent's kick from behind with the "***Black Dragon***

[I] *"Overhanging Fist"* (掛拳, Mandarin: *GUA QUAN*, Cantonese: *GWA KYUN*) - blow (or a block) with the back side of the fist and (or) the outer side of the forearm delivered from up to down. The fist moves from the shoulder level to the waist, making a semi-circle in the vertical plane **[index, p. 222]**.

[II] *"Throwing Fist"* (拋拳, Mandarin: *PAO QUAN,* Cantonese: *PAAU KYUN*) — a blow with the back of a fist, from down to up. The arm is almost completely straightened at the elbow joint. The movement starts from the hip and is reinforced due to a turn of the body. Another arm naturally draws down and backwards. This technique can serve as a block: in this case, the outer surface of a forearm is used. The final phase of the blow is shown in **Fig. 78**, **[index, p. 226]**.

[III] *"Beat the Drum With a Stone Pestle"* (碌鼓搥, Mandarin: *LU GU CHUI,* Cantonese: *LUK GU CEOI*) — a series of two blows performed one after the other, without a pause; first, an *"Overhanging Fist"* (掛拳) blow is delivered, followed immediately by a *"Throwing Fist"* (拋拳) blow **[index, p. 215]**.

Whipping Its Tail" technique: both forearms sweep from left to right, at waist level. It is the double *GWA* ("*Overhanging Blow*"). You look backward over your right shoulder. Practically, the block is made with the outer side of the right forearm, the left arm only reinforces the movement. This position is not shown in the book, but its image is in Lam Sai Wing's book ***"Tiger and Crane"***, **Fig. 79**.

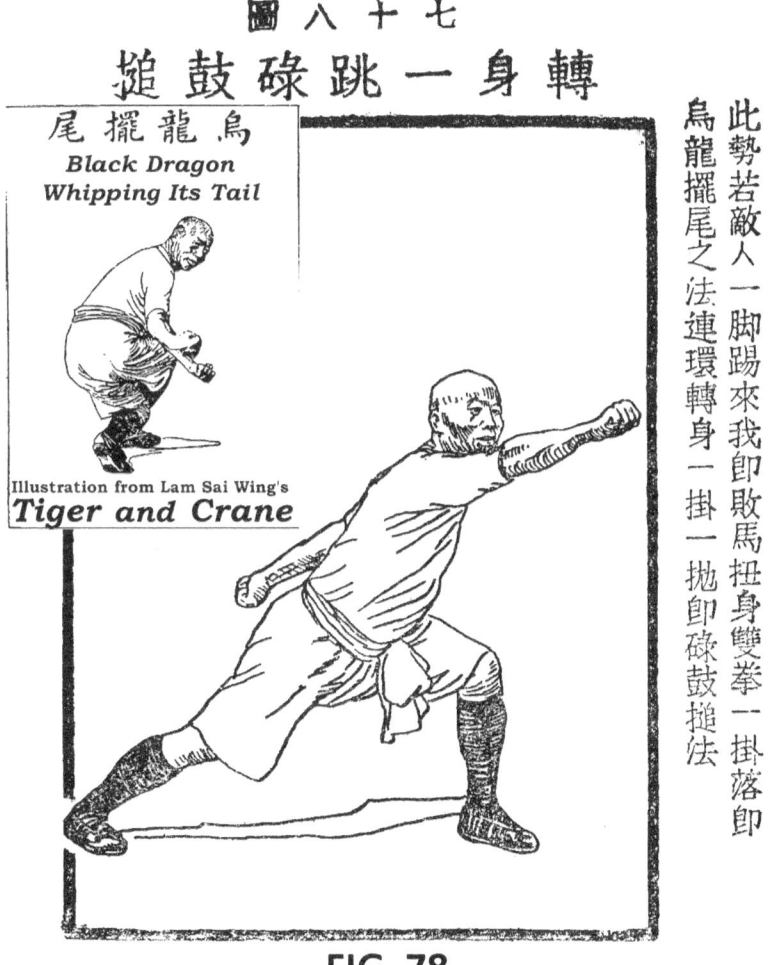

圖八十七

轉身一跳碌鼓搥

烏龍擺尾
**Black Dragon
Whipping Its Tail**

Illustration from Lam Sai Wing's
Tiger and Crane

此勢若敵人一脚踢來我即敗馬扭身雙拳一掛落即
烏龍擺尾之法連環轉身一掛一拋即碌鼓搥法

FIG. 78

Without pausing in the position "***Black Dragon Whipping Its Tail***," turn (without lifting your feet) 180 degrees counterclockwise and assume the ***SEI PING MAA*** ("*Horse Stance*"). Then, perform a low jump in place on both legs and land in the same position. Then, transition to the left-handed *JI NG MAA* (*"Bow and Arrow"*) stance. As you transition, deliver the **GWA** and **PAAU** strikes, which naturally follow one another, following the movement of your body. The final phase (**PAAU** blow) is shown in **Fig. 78**; it is delivered with your right arm, and the **GWA** blow is delivered with the left one.

七十九　出右攻迫左側掌

CHU YOU GONG PO ZUO QE ZHANG (Mandarin)
CHEUT JAU GUNG BIK JO JAK JEUNG (Cantonese)

79. Step to the Right, Blocking the Attack, Left Side Palm.

Blocking an attack with a bridge-arm is used when an opponent approaches and strikes me in the upper body. I immediately block their strike with my forearm and immediately counter with a "Side Palm"[I] blow. This blow is delivered with the heel of the palm, simultaneously with a step forward. This technique is called "Hide the Flower in the Sleeve."[II]

Commentaries: After performing the ***"Beat the Drum With a Stone Pestle"*** technique (**Fig. 78**), turn your torso 90 degrees to the right and assume the ***SEI PING MAA*** (*"Horse Stance"*) stance. Simultaneously, perform a block with your right forearm from bottom to top, parrying the opponent's strike to your head (**Fig. 79**). Without stopping, make a small half step

---

[I] *"Side Palm"* (側掌, Mandarin: **QE ZHANG**, Cantonese: **JAK JEUNG**) - a blow with the heel of an open palm, fingers turned outward (another name: ***"Hide the Flower in the Sleeve"***, 袖裏藏花), **[index, p. 224]**.

[II] *"Hide the Flower in the Sleeve"* (袖裏藏花, Mandarin: **XIU GUO ZONG HUA**, Cantonese: **ZAU GWO CONG FAA**) - a blow with the heel of an open hand, fingers turned outward, Fig. 80, **[index, p. 219]**.

with your right foot, transition to the right-handed *JI NG MAA* ("*Bow and Arrow*") stance, and deliver the **"Hide the Flower in the Sleeve"** blow to an enemy's chest or ribs with the heel of your left palm.

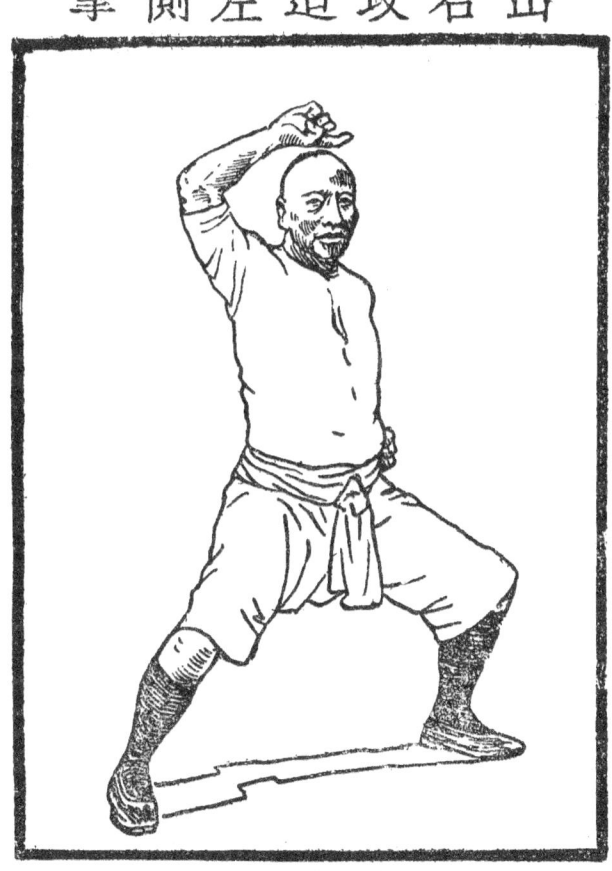

七十九圖
出右攻迫左側掌

攻迫橋手倘敵人由頭部打來我即用攻迫手招之連
用側掌打出此掌由夾底打出即袖裏藏花之法

FIG. 79

八十　左馬攻迫側掌來

ZUO MA GONG PO QE ZHANG LAI (Mandarin)
JO MAA GUNG BIK JAK JEUNG LOI (Cantonese)

80. Repeat in the Left-Hand Stance: Blocking the Attack, Side Palm.

"Bridge Blocking the Attack" - this technique is performed in the Stable Horse Riding Stance[I], which immediately transforms into the JI NG MAA stance. At this moment, a "Side Palm" blow is delivered to the enemy's side or ribs, at the level of his waist. The opponent manages to step back and avoid my blow. He immediately lifts his foot for a kick, and without hesitation, I advance forward in the JI NG MAA[II] stance and, by a covering motion of my palm from above, near his knee, stop the kick.

Commentaries: Here, the previous technique is done to the other side: from the previous position (**Fig. 79**), take a small step forward and to the left with your left foot and assume the ***"Stable Horse Riding Stance."*** Simultaneously, perform a block with your left forearm from bottom to top, parrying the opponent's strike to your head. Without stopping, make a small half step with your left foot, transition to the left-handed ***JI NG MAA*** (*"Bow and Arrow"*) stance, and deliver the ***"Hide the Flower in the Sleeve"*** blow to an enemy's chest or ribs with the heel of your right palm (**Fig. 80**). Then proceed to the next technique (**Fig. 81**).

[I] *"Stable Horse Riding Stance"* (四平八分馬, Mandarin: *SEI PING BA FEN MA*, Cantonese: *SEI PING BAAT FAN MAA*) – literally: *"Four Levels Eight Parts Horse Stance"* - lower *"Horse Stance"*, i.e., the feet are widespread, the center of gravity is situated low (Fig. 79), **[see index, p. 225]**.

[II] *JI NG MAA* (子午馬, Mandarin: *ZI WU MA*, Cantonese: *JI NG MAA*) - known in the modern *WUSHU* as the stance *"Bow and Arrow"* (Fig. 80). The term *"MAA"* is used in the meaning "a stance" here **[see index, p. 220]**.

左馬攻迫側掌來

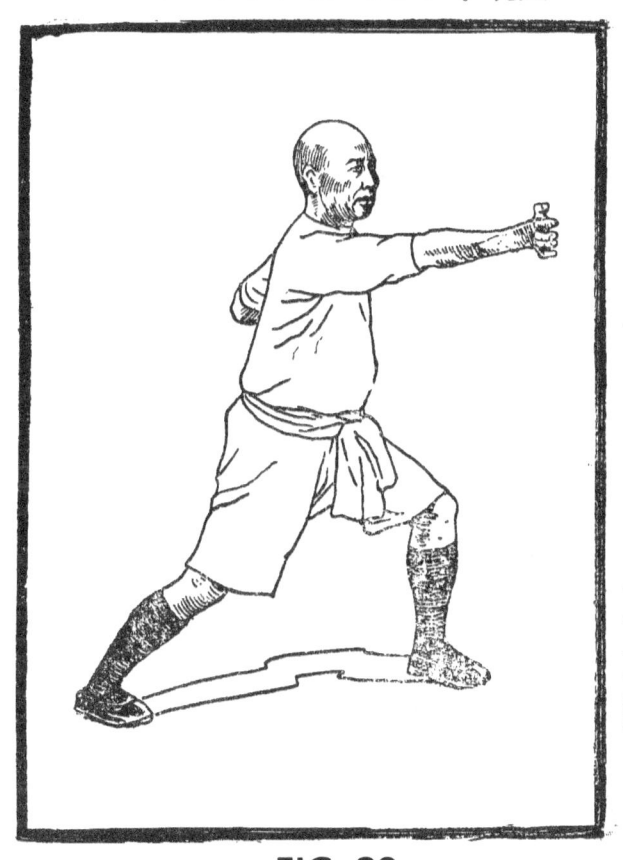

攻橋之法須用四平八分馬連轉子午馬側掌打敵人
腰部敵人連環回身起脚我卽上馬用冚手伏他膝部

FIG. 80

八十一 上右子午冚膀手

SHANG YOU ZI WU KAN BANG SHOU (Mandarin)
SOENG JAU JI NG KAM BONG SAU (Cantonese)

81. Step Forward Into a Right-Handed JI NG, Covering followed by the Arm Like a Wing.

The "Covering Wing"[I] technique is used if the enemy attacks with a kick. I immediately apply downward pressure with my hand, covering the attacking leg near the knee. The opponent follows up with a mid-level punch, which I immediately counter with the "Single Arm like a Wing"[II] technique. Then, without stopping or interrupting my movement, I transition to the "Lock the Iron Gate with a Bolt Weighing 1000 Jin"[III] technique.

Commentaries: From the previous position (**Fig. 80**), make a step with your right foot forward and take the position shown in **Fig. 81**. It is a blocking of the enemy's kick. If the enemy continues his attack with a fist blow at the middle level, shift your body weight to your back (left) foot and take the right-

---

[I] *"Covering Wing"* (冚膀, Mandarin: *KAN BANG* , Cantonese: *KAM BONG*) - blocking a strike with the hand (palm), usually from top to bottom, with a "pressing" or "slapping" motion (**Fig. 81**) **[index, p. 216]**.

[II] *"Single Arm like a Wing"* (單膀手, Mandarin: *DAN BANG SHOU*, Cantonese: *DAAN BONG SAU*) - a forearm block **[see index, p. 224]**.

[III] *"Lock the Iron Gate with a Bolt Weighing 1000 Jin"* (鐵門閂槌千斤, Mandarin: *TIE MEN SHUAN CHUI QIAN JIN*, Cantonese: - *TIT MUN SAAN CHEUI CIN GAN*) - a technique that has various applications, which are described later in this book (see **Fig. 82**), as well as in **Lam Sai Wing**'s book "Tiger and Crane". In this case, it refers to a simultaneous punch with both fists, from the bottom up, with an upward movement, aimed at the opponent's stomach and neck (or chin). *Jin* (Cantonese: *Gan*, 斤) is a traditional Chinese unit for weight. One *Jin* is approximately equal to 1.316 *lb* (600 *g*) **[see index, p. 221]**.

handed **_"Hanging Foot Stance"_** (_"The Cat's Stance"_). At the same time, execute a "soft" deflecting block from outside to inside with your right forearm: your arm is bent at the elbow, the forearm is vertical, the palm is open, and the fingers are directed down. The left palm is located near the right shoulder and turned to the right.

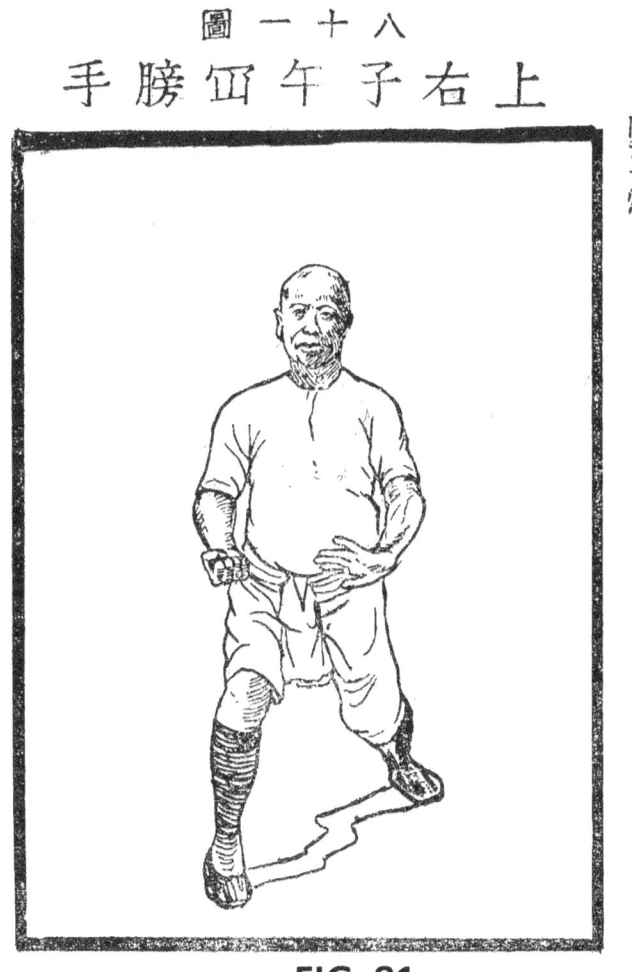

圖一十八

手膀𨂂午子右上

𨂂膀之法敵人用腳踢來我即用手佝他膝部他連環
用中拳打來我即用單膀手法扲之連用鉄門門千斤
墜之法

FIG. 81

Catch the enemy's arm with both hands, sharply jerk it towards you and downwards, at the same time make a step forward with your right foot and return to the initial right-handed stance _**JI NG MAA**_ _('Bow and Arrow')_. At this moment, deliver the simultaneous punches with both fists, from the bottom, with an upward movement, aimed at the opponent's stomach and neck (or chin). This is the technique *"Lock the Iron Gate with a Bolt Weighing 1000 Jin"* (**Fig. 82**).

八十二　千斤一墜鐵門閂

QIAN JIN YI ZHUI TIE MEN SHUAN (Mandarin)
CIN GAN JAT ZEOI TIT MUN SAAN (Cantonese)

82. Drop a 1000 Jin and Lock the Iron Gate.

If the opponent attacks me with a punch to the mid-level, I parry his attack with the "Single Arm Like a Wing" technique. If the opponent follows up with a kick, I will drop a 1000 Jin and crush his attack, and then, without stopping, attack them with the "Locking the Iron Gate" technique.

Commentaries: You parried the enemy's punch with the ***"Single Arm like a Wing,"*** but the enemy continues the attack and immediately kicks. Shift your weight to your back (left) foot and enter ***"Hanging Foot Stance"*** (*"The Cat's Stance"*). Simultaneously, pull both fists toward your left shoulder, and from there, without stopping the movement, immediately and sharply lower both forearms to waist level. It is a block against a kick: the forearms are horizontal, the wrists are bent inward, and the backs of the fists are facing down. Blocking is performed with the outside of the forearms, from top to bottom. This is the first phase of the ***"Lock the Iron Gate with a Bolt Weighing 1000 Jin"*** technique. Without pausing in this position, step forward with your right foot and return to the starting ***JI NG MAA*** (*"Bow and Arrow"*) *stance*. As you enter the stance, deliver the simultaneous punches with both fists, from the bottom, with an upward movement, aimed at the opponent's stomach and neck (or chin). It is the second (and final) phase of the technique ***"Lock the Iron Gate with a Bolt Weighing 1000 Jin"*** (**Fig. 82**).

千斤一墜鐵門閂

此勢倘敵人中拳打來我用單膀手法招之他用腳打來我用千斤墜破之連用鐵門閂法攻他

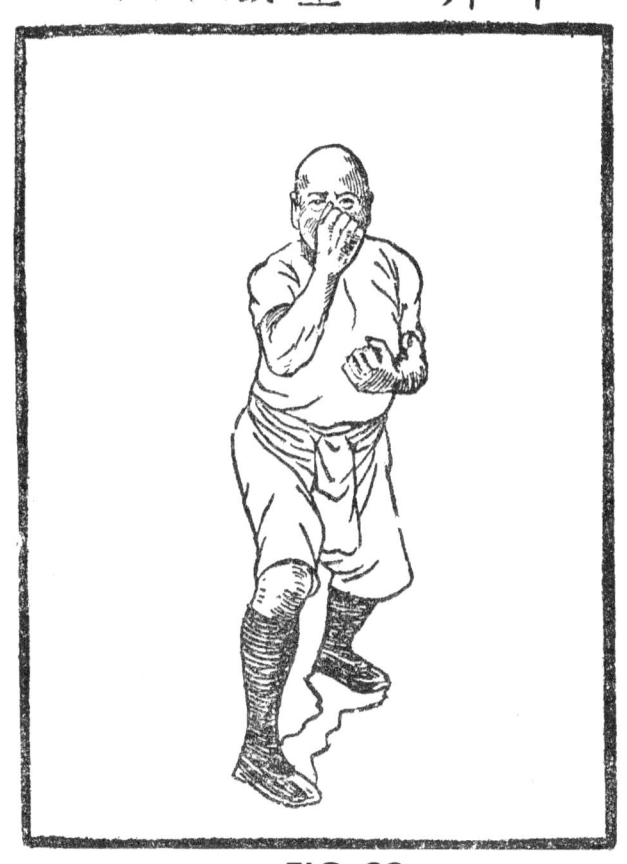

FIG. 82

八十三　跳馬猛弓射箭搥

TIAO MA MENG GONG SHE JIAN CHUI (Mandarin)
TIU MAA MANG GUNG SE JIN CEOI (Cantonese)

83. Jump, Stance MAA, Draw the Bow and Shoot the Arrow.

To deliver the "Draw the Bow and Shoot the Arrow"[I] blow, you must squat down into a low "Four Levels Eight Parts Horse Stance"[II]. Your shoulders and the striking arm are in the same (horizontal) line: this position resembles the outline of the character for "Sun" (日). If the enemy evades and attempts to counterattack, stun them with a continuous series of "Uninterrupted Punches like Rockets"[III], transitioning seamlessly to the "Hook Spring Leg"[IV] technique — this is the "sweeping" technique.

[I] *"Draw the Bow and Shoot the Arrow"* (猛弓射箭, Mandarin: *MENG GONG SHE JIAN*, Cantonese: *MANG GUNG SE JIN*) - see text and commentaries to Fig. 83, **[index, p. 223]**.

[II] *"Stable Horse Riding Stance"* (四平八分馬, Mandarin: *SEI PING BA FEN MA*, Cantonese: *SEI PING BAAT FAN MAA*) – literally: *"Four Levels Eight Parts Horse Stance"* - lower *"Horse Stance"*, i.e., the feet are widespread, the center of gravity is situated low **(Fig. 83)**, **[see index, p. 225]**.

[III] *"Uninterrupted Punches like Rockets"* or *"Fists like Rockets Strike one after another"* (火箭連環拳, Mandarin: *HUO JIAN LIAN HUAN QUAN*, Cantonese: *FO JIN LIN WAAN KYUN*) - a rapid succession of punches, following each other without a break, like rain drumming on a roof **[see index, p. 227]**.

[IV] *"Hook Spring Leg"* (拘彈脚, Mandarin: *ZU TAN JIAO*, Cantonese: *KEOI TAAN GEUK*), the same as the *"Three-Star Hook Spring Leg"* (三星鉤彈腳, Mandarin: *SAN SING ZHU TAN JIAO*, Cantonese: *SAAM SING KAU TAAN GEUK*) - a low sweeping kick with the shin (lower shinbone), hooking and sweeping of the front-standing leg of the enemy, followed by a kick to the knee or ankle of his supporting leg or a reverse leg sweep **[see index, pp. 219, 226]**.

Commentaries: Change in a jump your position from the stance shown in **Fig. 82** into the ***SEI PING BAAT FAN MAA*** (*"Stable Horse Stance"*, **Fig. 83**). It allows avoiding a blow to your head or to your breast. When you jump, your right arm deflects the blow aside or grips the striking arm of the enemy with a subsequent jerk to yourself.

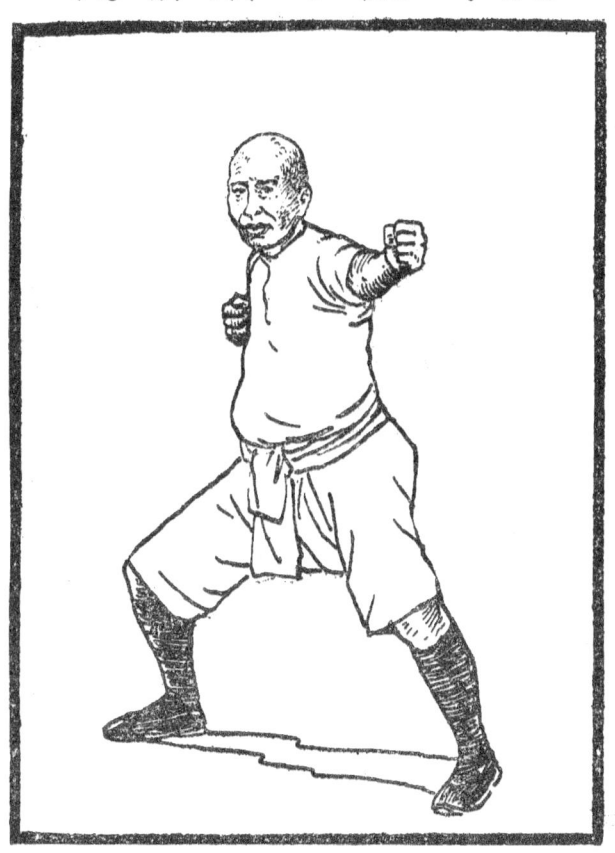

圖 三 十 八

搥箭射弓猛馬跳

猛弓射箭拳法低座四平八分馬單肩脾日字拳如搖
弓射箭一般打出他招我即用連環火箭拳再用扚
彈脚法扚之

FIG. 83

Deliver a blow with your left fist to an enemy's side at the moment of landing into the ***SEI PING BAAT FAN MAA*** stance, then turn to the ***JI NG MAA*** (*"Bow and Arrow"*) stance and punch with your right fist. After it, "hack" the enemy's front leg with your right shin (lower shinbone) and immediately deliver a "cutting" kick to the knee or ankle of his supporting leg with the side of your right foot, or use a reverse leg sweep. All movements must be done quickly, without pauses.

八十四　抅彈一迫黑虎爪
ZU TAN YI PO HEI HU ZHAO (Mandarin)
KEOI TAAN JAT BIK HAAK FU ZAAU (Cantonese)

84. Sweeping and Cutting, Approaching and Black Tiger Claw.

"Hook Spring" is a hooking, followed by a reverse sweeping. These actions are seamlessly transformed into the "Black Tiger Claws"[1] technique. This technique requires close contact with the opponent. You must decisively advance forward, step by step, and attack.

Commentaries: After finishing the *"Hook Spring Leg"* technique, step forward with your right foot into a right-handed **JI NG MAA** (*"Bow and Arrow"*) stance and perform the *"Black Tiger Claw"* technique: the left hand in the "tiger's claw" position delivers a blow, the right arm (the hand is also in the "tiger's claw" position) protects the stomach and the breast from a possible counterattack (**Fig. 84**). Here the author stresses that it is necessary to combine actions of arms and legs skillfully, to advance resolutely with changing levels and directions of attacks, to suppress the enemy with a series of blows.

---

[1] *"Black Tiger Claw"* (黑虎爪, Mandarin: *HEI HU ZHAO*, Cantonese: *HAAK FU ZAAU*) - a strike with a hand in the position *"Tiger Claw"* to the enemy's face with a subsequent grip and a squeeze, or ripping motion from top to bottom (**Fig. 84**). This technique and its combat application are described in detail by Lam Sai Wing in *Tiger and Crane*, Fig. 94, **[see index, p. 215]**.

扚彈一迫黑虎爪

扚有扚彈有彈連轉黑虎爪法此勢須用交加手無論如何進馬步步攻之

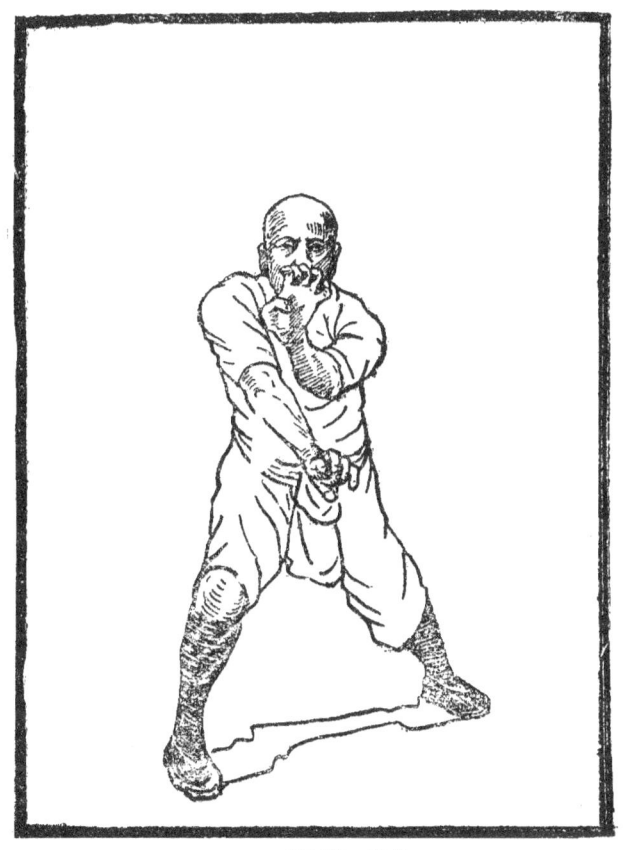

FIG. 84

八十五　退馬金龍爪獻來

TUI MA JIN LONG ZHAO XIAN LAI (Mandarin)
TEOI MAA GAM LUNG ZAAU HIN LOI (Cantonese)

85. Retreat in Position, Golden Dragon Presents Its Claws.

If an enemy approaches from behind and strikes me, I immediately retreat into a defensive stance, both my hands in the position "Claws" move back and parry his attack. It is the "Golden Dragon Presents Its Claws"[I] technique. I do not stop and continue to turn my body, use one of my arms in the position "Bridge", advance in the stance, and deliver a fist blow with the other arm.

Commentaries: From the position shown in **Fig. 84**, transfer your body weight to your front (right) foot and rotate your upper body 90 degrees to the right, assuming the position shown in **Fig. 85**. Simultaneously, both forearms (hands in the **"Claws"** position) sweep to the right, deflecting the opponent's strike. Without lingering in the position shown in **Fig. 85**, turn anticlockwise around 180 degrees and take the **SEI PING MAA** (*"Horse Stance"*). Parry a possible second attack to your head or to your breast with the left "bridge" (**Fig. 86**). Then immediately deliver a straight punch with your right fist to the middle level. While delivering a punch, turn your body to the left-handed stance **JI NG MAA** (*"Bow and Arrow"*) to make the blow stronger.

[I] **"Golden Dragon Presents Its Claws"** (金龍爪獻, Mandarin: **JIN LONG ZHAO XIAN**, Cantonese: **GAM LUNG ZAAU HIN**) - turn toward the attacking opponent with a sweeping block with both forearms in a horizontal plane; hands in a "claw" position; the twisting force of the lower back is used, which enhances the blocking motion of the forearms (Fig. 85) **[index, p. 218]**.

退馬金龍爪獻來

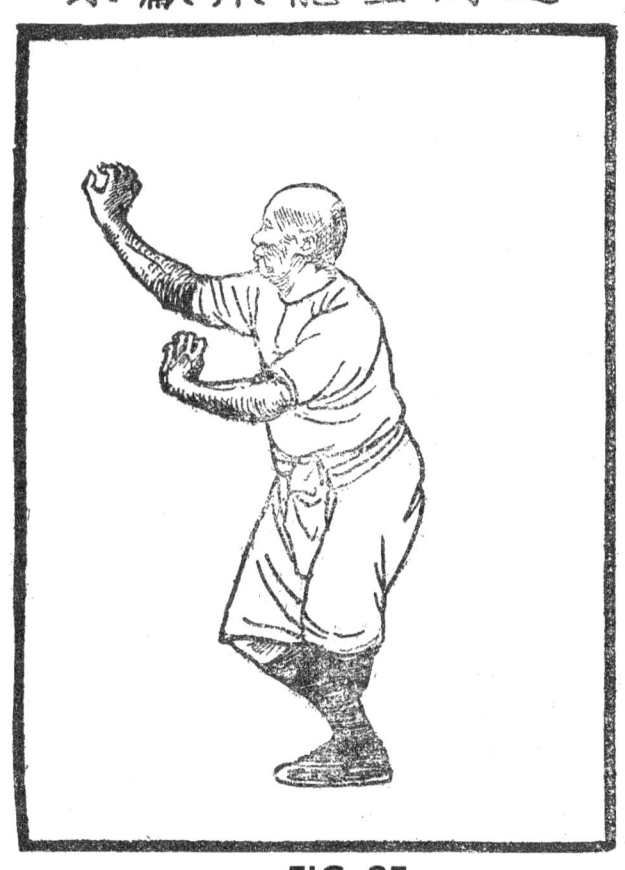

FIG. 85

如敵人由後打來我即退馬將雙爪歸後招之即金龍
獻爪之法連轉身一橋手進馬一拳打出

八十六　轉身一橋搥打出

ZHUAN SHEN YI QIAO CHUI DA CHU (Mandarin)
JYUN SAN JAT KIU CEOI DAA CHEUT (Cantonese)

86. Turn Around, One Bridge, One Straight Punch.

If the enemy delivers a fist blow to the middle part of my body, I use the "Hanging Foot Stance"[I], "Pushing Elbow"[II], "Hand Coiling Around a Branch"[III], and pull his arm toward me. Then I immediately deliver a straight punch to his side at waist level or apply the "Hide the Flower in the Sleeve"[IV] technique.

Commentaries: The title of this figure and the position (technique) shown in the **Fig. 86** refer to the previous actions described in the text and comments for **Fig. 85**. The text for this figure describes the subsequent actions shown in **Fig. 87** and **Fig. 88**.

[I] *"Hanging Foot Stance"* (馬吊腳, Mandarin: *MA DIAO JIAO*, Cantonese: *MAA DIU GEUK*) - known in modern *WUSHU* as the *"Cat's Stance"* (**Fig. 26**). The term *"MAA"* is used in the meaning "a stance" here **[index p. 219]**.

[II] *"Pushing Elbow"* (迫睜, Mandarin: *PO ZHENG*, Cantonese: *BIK ZAANG*) - using the elbow to block mid- and upper-level strikes; the elbow can be pushed forward to defend against a straight blow (and damage to the opponent's striking limb), or the elbow can be used in a vertical or diagonal motion to block strikes coming from different angles (**Fig. 87**) **[index, p. 223]**.

[III] *"Hand Coiling Around a Branch"* (纏枝手, Mandarin: *CHAN ZHI SHOU*, Cantonese: *CIN ZI SAU*) - a deflecting block with a possible subsequent grab of the opponent's arm; performed by "coiling" hand movement around the forearm of the opponent's attacking arm **[index p. 218]**.

[IV] *"Hide the Flower in the Sleeve"* (袖裏藏花, Mandarin: *XIU GUO ZONG HUA*, Cantonese: *ZAU GWO CONG FAA*) - a blow with the heel of an open hand, fingers turned outward, Fig. 80, **[index, p. 219]**.

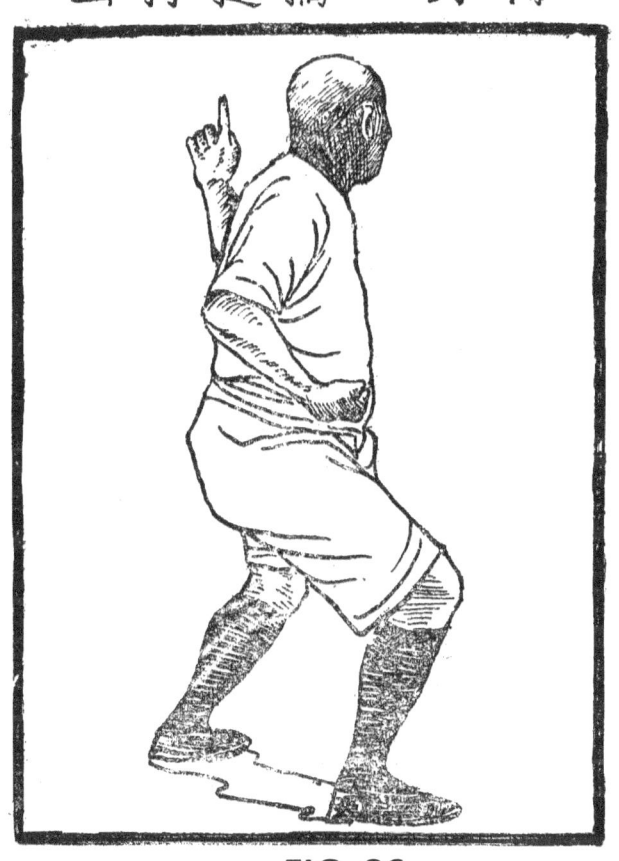

FIG. 86

若他人一拳中部打來我用吊腳迫脛纏枝手伏他脛
連用拳打他腰部即袖裏藏花之法

八十七　吊左纏枝一搥來

DIAO ZUO CHAN ZHI YI CHUI LAI (Mandarin)
DIU JO CIN ZI JAT CEOI LOI (Cantonese)

87. Hang on the Left, Coiling Around a Branch, Follow With a Punch.

The "Hand Coiling Around a Branch" technique is used in the following situation: for example, an opponent approaches and punches me. I immediately use "Pushing Elbow" and immediately follow it with "Hand Coiling Around a Branch." There's a risk of the enemy feinting and trying to lure you into a trap, so immediately follow up with "Soul-Returning Hand."[I]

Commentaries: From the left-handed *JI NG MAA* (*"Bow and Arrow"*) stance, step your right foot forward and to the right (at a 45-degree angle) and transition to the right-handed *"Hanging Foot Stance"* (*"Cat's Stance"*). Bend your right arm and, with your right elbow, from the outside in, block the opponent's strike; your right hand in a position *"Claw"* (*"Pushing Elbow,"* **Fig. 87**). Don't linger in this position. Your right hand moves to the right and down, then to the left and up in a circular motion, as if you were "coiling" the opponent's attacking arm, and grab it with your right hand from above at the elbow or forearm, then pressing down and pulling it toward you (*"Hand Coiling Around a Branch"*). Simultaneously with the jerk, step forward with your right foot into a right-sided *JI NG MAA* (*"Bow and Arrow"*) stance and deliver a straight punch with your left fist to the enemy's side. It is the *"Soul Returning Hand"* technique. This combination is then performed on the other side, starting from

---

[I] *"Soul-Returning Hand"* (還魂手, Mandarin: *HUAN HUN SHOU*, Cantonese: *WAAN WAN SAU*) - a straight punch with the rear fist in the *JI NG MAA* (*"Bow and Arrow"*) position, Fig. 88, **[index, p. 224]**.

a left-handed ***"Hanging Foot Stance"*** (*"Cat's Stance"*), so **Fig. 88** depicts a punch with the right fist.

圖七十八

來搥一枝纏左吊

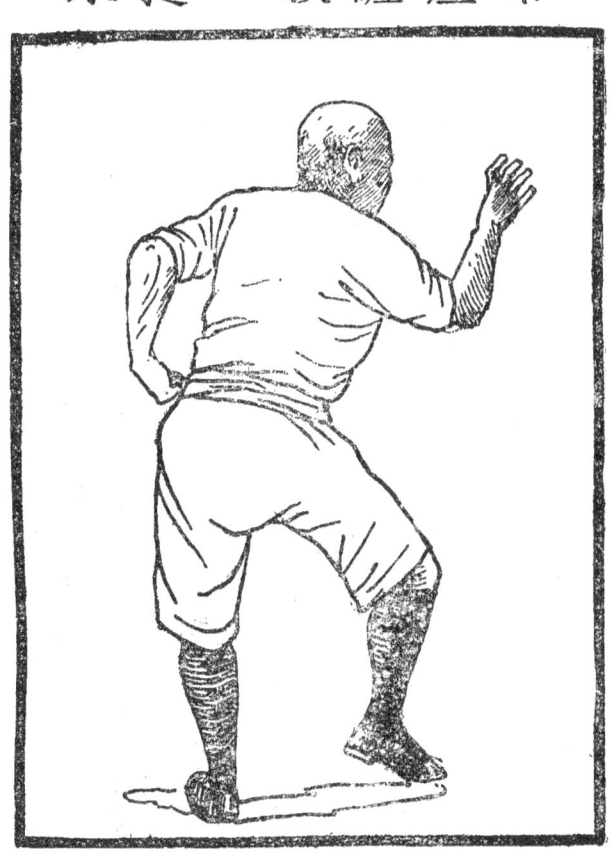

他若逢伏胛即須用還魂手法

逢纏枝手法如敵人一拳打來我即用迫胛纏枝手伏

FIG. 87

八十八　左右連環各一勻
ZUO YOU LIAN HUAN GE YI YUN (Mandarin)
JO JAU LIN WAAN GOK JAT WAN (Cantonese)

88. Left and Right, Continuously, Equally on Each Side.

When using the "Pushing Elbow", it is necessary to be in the position of the "Hanging Foot Stance", then use the method "Hand Coiling Around a Branch" and eliminate an enemy's attack by applying force to his elbow. After it, without stopping, it is necessary to deliver a fist blow. If the enemy uses the "Pushing Elbow" technique against me and tries to deliver a fist blow, I immediately advance in the MAA position, use the "Black Tiger Claw"[I] technique, and overwhelm the enemy.

Commentaries: Here, the above-mentioned combination is executed on the other side. If the enemy tries to use a similar technique against you, it is necessary to lower yourself to a stable stance ***JI NG MAA*** (*"Bow and Arrow"*), to parry his attack with the front arm and to deliver a blow with the "claws" of the rear hand to the face or the throat of the enemy (see **Fig. 84**).

[I] **"Black Tiger Claw"** (黑虎爪, Mandarin: **HEI HU ZHAO**, Cantonese: **HAAK FU ZAAU**) - a strike with a hand in the position **"Tiger Claw"** to the enemy's face with a subsequent grip and a squeeze, or ripping motion from top to bottom (**Fig. 84**). This technique and its combat application are described in detail by **Lam Sai Wing** in *Tiger and Crane*, **Fig. 94**, [index, p. 215].

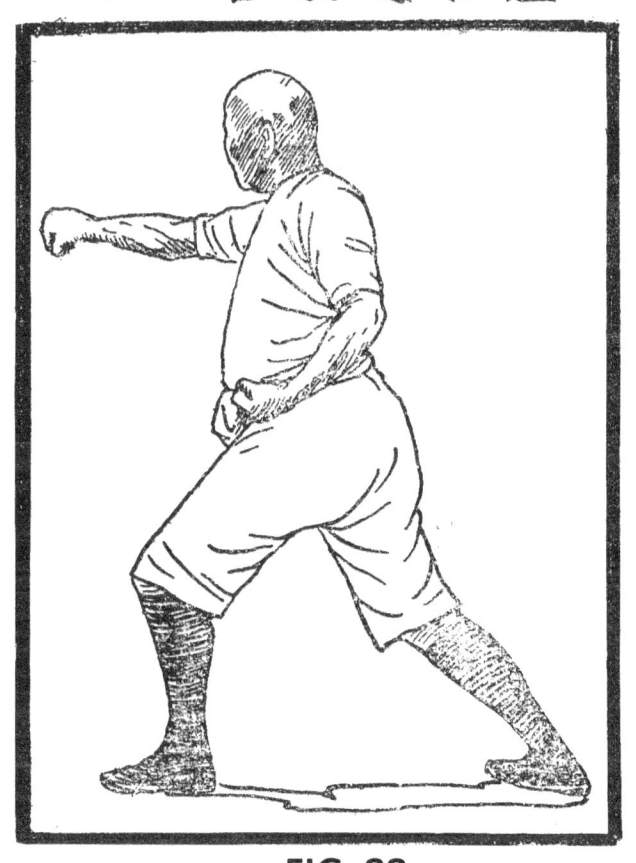

八十八圖

左右連環各一勻

逢迫脛須用吊腳纏枝手伏他脛部連環一拳若他人
伏我脛一拳打來我即上馬連用黑虎爪伏他

FIG. 88

八十九　蝶掌一攋分左右

DIE ZHANG YI LA FEN ZUO YOU (Mandarin)
DIP JEUNG JAT LAAP FAN JO JAU (Cantonese)

89. Palms Like Butterflies, Collect and Separate, Left and Right.

If an enemy attacks me with a punch, I immediately counter with the "Butterfly Palms"ᴵ. The enemy responds with "Butterfly Palms" too. If the attacking "Butterfly Palms" are countered with the "Butterfly Palms", the one with the greater strength wins. If the enemy is stronger than I am and suppresses my attack by force, I immediately proceed to the technique "Turn and Divide, Penetrate with Hands"ᴵᴵ and break him.

Commentaries: The technique *"Palms like Butterflies"* is successively executed to the left and to the right side. The nuances of performing the *"Palms like Butterflies"* and *"Turn and Divide, Penetrate with Hands"* techniques, and their combat applications, are discussed in the comments to **Figs. 9**, **52**, and **53**.

ᴵ *"Palms like Butterflies"* (蝶掌, Mandarin: *DIE ZHANG*, Cantonese: *DIP JEUNG*) - circular block with both palms in the frontal plane, followed by a simultaneous blow with open palms at two levels, the fingers of the upper palm are directed upwards, the fingers of the lower palm are directed downwards (**Figs. 52, 63, 66, 89**), **[see index, p. 223]**.

ᴵᴵ *"Turn and Divide, Penetrate with Hands"* (轉分漏手, Mandarin: *ZHUAN FEN LOU SHOU*, Cantonese: *JYUN FAN LAU SAU*) - see commentaries on **p. 44**, **[see index, p. 226]**.

八十九圖

蝶掌一攤分左右

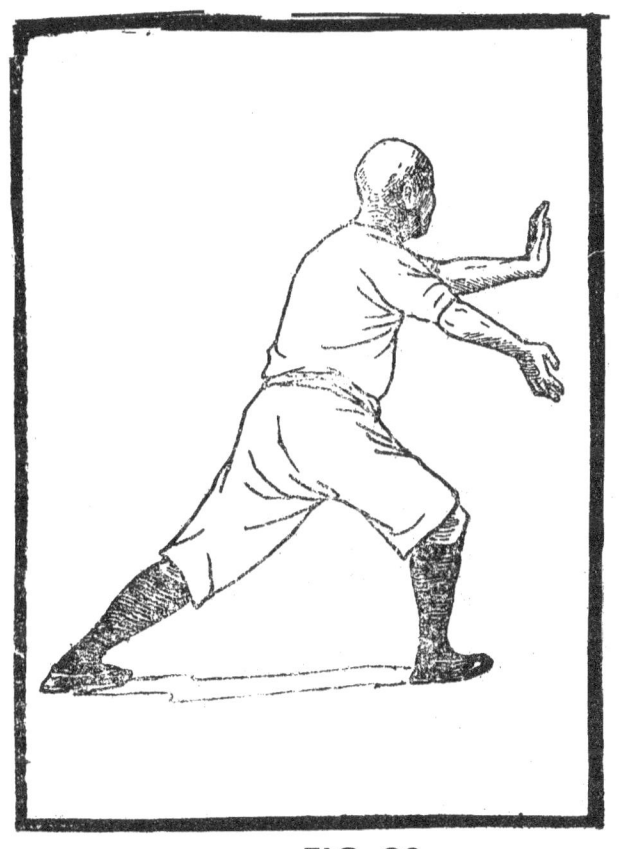

FIG. 89

倘敵人一拳打來我即用蝶掌招之他亦用蝶掌招我
所謂蝶掌來蝶掌送力大者則勝力弱者敗若他力大
我即用分漏手法破之

九十　三星連環黑虎爪

SAN XING LIAN HUAN HEI HU ZHAO (Mandarin)
SAAM SING LIN WAAN HAAK FU ZAAU (Cantonese)

90. Three Star in a Row, and Black Tiger Claws.

The continuous "Three Star" series is a series of successive strikes of GWA[I], ZAAK[II], and then KAM DENG[III]. It is a downward blow, like hammering a nail. A continuous chain of strikes, one after another: GWAA, ZAAK, and KAM DENG – this is the "Three Star" technique. If my opponent attacks me with a punch to my middle level, I use a series of GWAA, ZAAK, and KAM DENG strikes. I attack continuously, advancing step by step, and immediately transition to the "Black Tiger Claw" technique.

Commentaries: After performing the ***"Palms like Butterflies"*** technique left and right, step forward with your right foot into the ***SEI PING MAA*** (*"Horse Stance"*). Simultaneously, execute a ***GWA*** strike with your right arm. In

---

[I] *"Overhanging Fist"* (掛拳, Mandarin: *GUA QUAN*, Cantonese: *GWA KYUN*) - blow (or a block) with the back side of the fist and (or) the outer side of the forearm delivered from up to down. The fist moves from the shoulder level to the waist, making a semi-circle in the vertical plane **[index, p. 222]**.

[II] *"Pressing Fist"* (責拳, Mandarin: *ZE QUAN*, Cantonese: *ZAAK KYUN*), also known as the *"Hammer Fist"* - blow (or a block) with the forearm and (or) the bottom of the fist, the part near the little finger; delivered from top to bottom **[index, p. 223]**.

[III] *"Slap With the Palm to Drive a Nail"* (山釘拳, Mandarin: *KAN DING QUAN*, Cantonese: *KAM DENG KYUN*) - a blow (or block) with the heel of a clenched fist; delivered from top to bottom, or from top to bottom diagonally, or in horizontal plane **[index, p. 224]**. There is an exercise in the hard branch of *Shaolin Qi Gong* for nailing with a hand, which probably gave the name to this technique: a big nail, abutting the center of a palm with its head and being held with the extreme phalanges of the middle and fourth finger, is driven into a board with one strike.

this combination, this is a block against a straight punch. Without interrupting the movement, pivot 90 degrees to the right to the right-sided stance *JI NG MAA* (*"Bow and Arrow"*) and immediately execute a *ZAAK* blow with your left forearm.

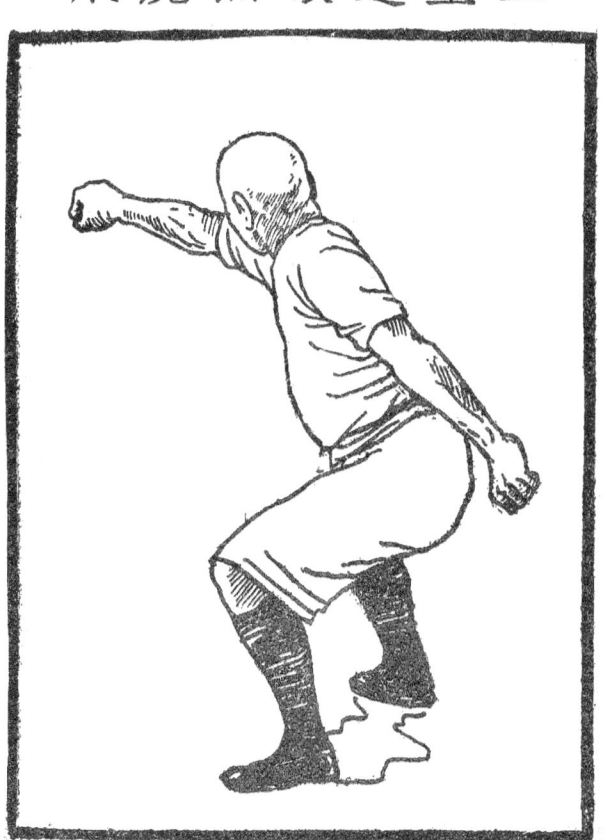

爪虎黑環連星三　　圖十九

連環三星用掛責拳落一釘連環掛冚釘拳之法如敵
人中拳打來我用掛責冚釘手步步進攻連轉黑虎爪
法

FIG. 90

In this case, this is a damaging blow to the elbow of the opponent's striking arm. Immediately, without stopping, execute a *KAM DENG* strike with your right hand. In this *TAO LU* (form), the *KAM DENG* strike is delivered vertically, from top to bottom. In real fighting use, the blow is delivered to the jaw angle, temple, or the back of the opponent's head. All three strikes are executed one after the other, without stopping.

九十一　轉身一橋又一搥

ZHUAN SHEN YI QIAO YOU YI CHUI (Mandarin)
JYUN SAN JAT KIU JAU JAT CEOI (Cantonese)

91. Turn Around, One Bridge and One Punch.

If the enemy attacks me from behind, I immediately turn and beat off his attack with a "Bridge", without stopping advance in the position, and deliver a fist blow to the central part of his breast. He parries my blow and attacks me with a fist blow again. In that case, I use a "Wing" to cover his arm and deliver a fist blow to him with the other hand.

Commentaries: Turn back and assume the **SEI PING MAA** (*"Horse Stance"*) , while simultaneously blocking the opponent's blow with your left forearm (橋,　**"Bridge"**), moving it transversely from the inside out (i.e., horizontally). Then, without stopping, take a small step forward with your left foot and assume the left-side *JI NG MAA* (*"Bow and Arrow"*) stance, delivering a straight blow ("**CHUI"**) to the enemy's chest with your right fist. If after parrying your blow, the enemy attacks you again, shift your body weight to your back leg and assume the left-side **"Hanging Foot Stance"** (*"Cat's Stance"*) at the same time, block the enemy's counterattack with your left arm in the "**Wing**" position and deliver a blow with your right fist (**Fig. 92**).

轉身一橋又一揰

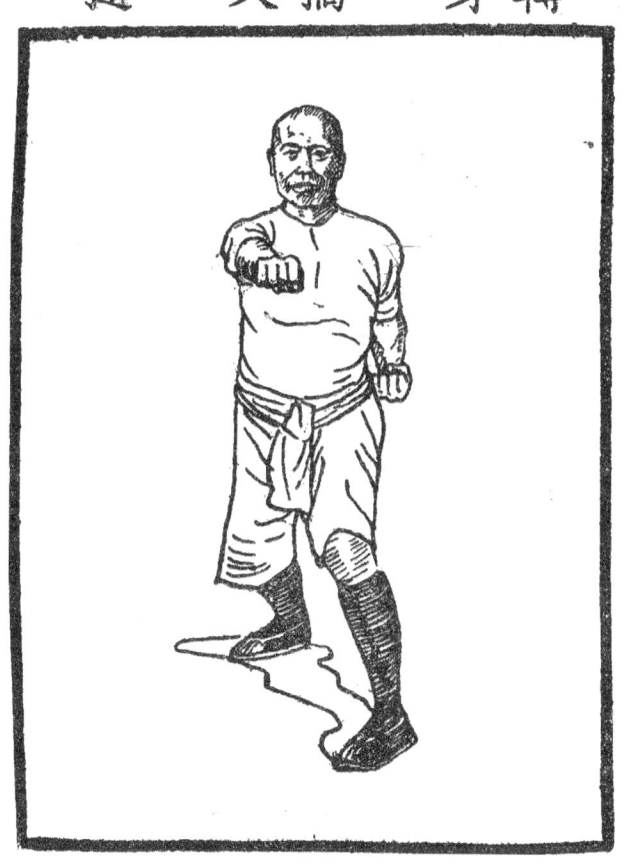

倘敵人由後打來我即轉身一橋連環進馬一拳打他
心胸他招我連用拳再來我用翅冚手一拳打他

FIG. 91

九十二　收拳見禮須吊腳

SHOU QUAN JIAN LI XU DIAO JIAO (Mandarin)
SAU KYUN GIN LAI SEOI DIU GEUK (Cantonese)

92. Pull Back Fist, Welcoming Ceremony in the Hanging Foot Stance.

Wing and Fist is the greeting ritual. It is necessary to assume the Hanging Foot Stance[I], retract your chest[II], and shape your hands for the greeting ritual. You show respect to your opponent with a slight smile, without malice or anger toward him, but rather by demonstrating humility and regard.

[I] *"Hanging Foot Stance"* (馬吊腳, Mandarin: *MA DIAO JIAO*, Cantonese: *MAA DIU GEUK*) - known in modern *WUSHU* as the *"Cat's Stance"* (**Fig. 26**). The term *"MAA"* is used in the meaning "a stance" here **[index p. 219]**.

[II] Requirements to the stance (**Fig. 92**): The shoulders are slightly advanced, the chest is slightly drawn inward ("**empty**"), the stomach is "**filled**" and tensed. As a result, *Qi* moves downward and concentrates in the *Dantian*. The center of your body weight is in a lower position, the position is stable, and your attention is concentrated. If the breast is "**filled**," i.e., thrust out, *Qi* is rushing up, the position is unstable, and it is difficult to achieve concentration.

收拳見禮須吊脚

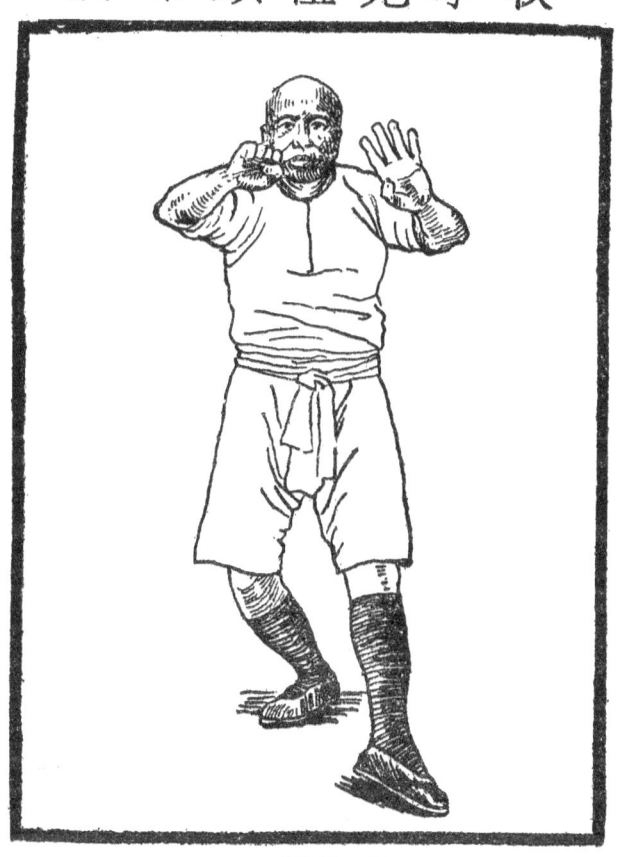

FIG. 92

起凹一拳即見禮一般須用吊脚收胸拱手見禮以微笑不可以怒氣對人以示謙讓

九十三　扭手收拳一鞠躬

NIU SHOU SHOU QUAN YI JU GONG (Mandarin)
NAU SAU SAU KYUN JAT GUK GUNG (Cantonese)

93. Clench Hands, Pull Back Fists, Bow as a Sign of Respect.

Clench your hands, pull your fists to the waist on both sides, pull in (retract) your chest, lower your shoulders, and make a respectful bow.

***

扭手收拳一鞠躬

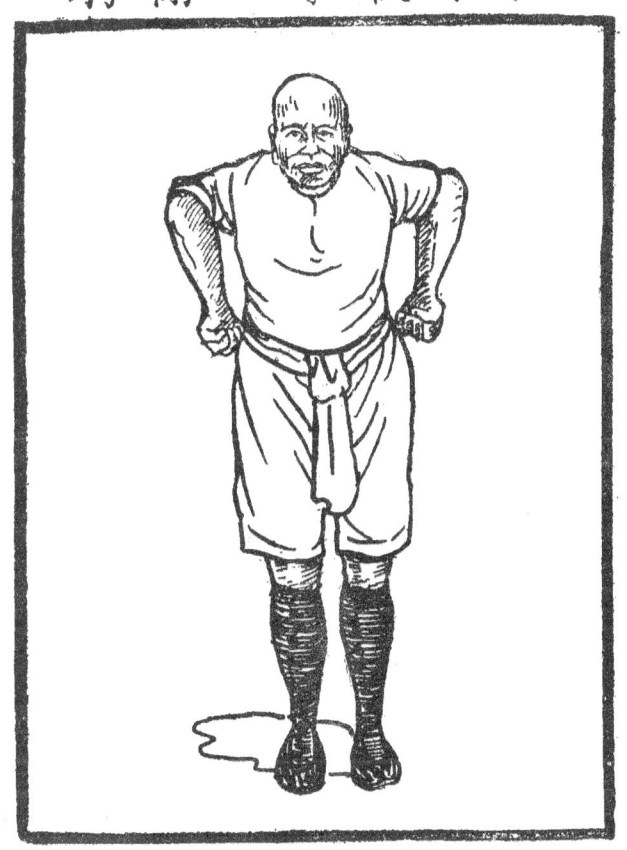

紐手收拳之法將拳收在腰傍收胸落膊一鞠躬

FIG. 93

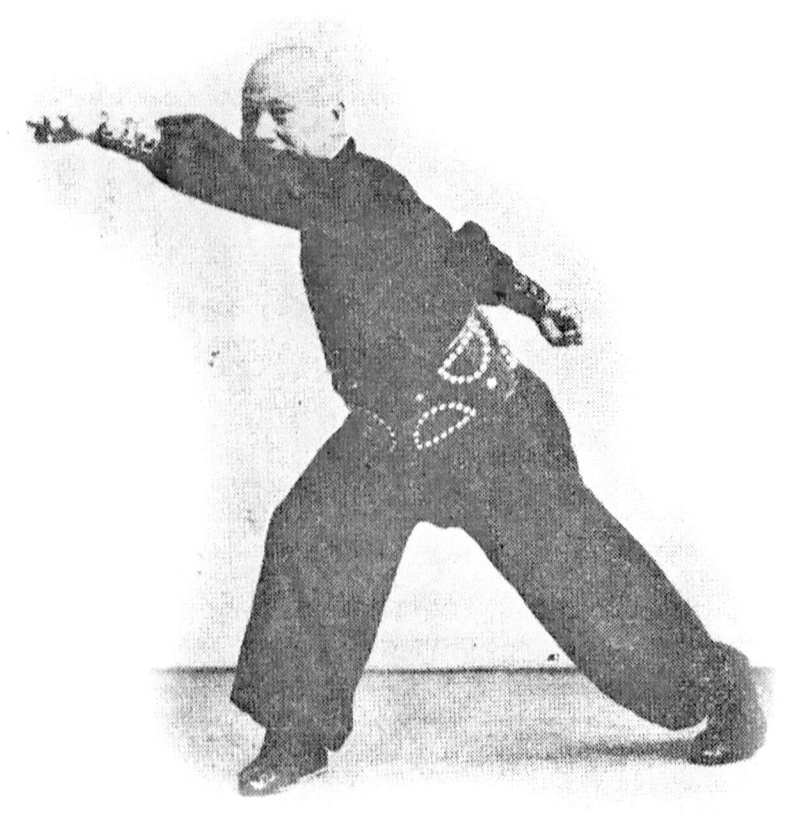

INDEX

A

"Arm Like a Wing" (膀手, Mandarin: *BANG SHOU*, Cantonese: *BONG SAU*), a forearm block **[pp. 64, 82, 108, 154, 222]**.

B

"Beat the Drum With a Stone Pestle" (碌鼓搥, Mandarin: *LU GU CHUI*, Cantonese: *LUK GU CEOI*) – a series of two blows performed one after the other, without a pause; first, an *"Overhanging Fist"* (掛拳) blow is delivered, followed immediately by a *"Throwing Fist"* (拋拳) blow **[pp. 182, 184]**.

"Black Dragon Whipping Its Tail" (烏龍擺尾, Mandarin: *WU LONG BAI WEI*, Cantonese: *WU LUNG BAAI MEI*) – sweeping block at mid-level with both forearms in the *Unicorn Step* position (see commentaries to **Fig. 77**). See also: Lam Sai Wing, *Tiger and Crane*, **Fig. 79**, **[pp. 180, 181, 182, 183]**.

"Black Tiger Claw" (黑虎爪, Mandarin: *HEI HU ZHAO*, Cantonese: *HAAK FU ZAAU*) - a blow with a hand in the position *"Tiger Claw"* to the enemy's face with a subsequent grip and a squeeze (**Fig. 84**), **[pp. 144, 145, 152, 154, 194, 202, 206]**. This technique and its combat application are described in detail by **Lam Sai Wing** in *Tiger and Crane*, **Fig. 94**. There is a method with a similar name *HEI HU SHOU* – *"Hand of Black Tiger"* among the called *"72 Secret Arts of Monks from the Shaolin Monastery"*. This method is intended to enhance the strength and hardness of fingers and nails, as well as the strength of a grip (Jin Jing Zhong. *Authentic Shaolin Heritage: Training Methods Of 72 Arts Of Shaolin*, Shaolin Kung Fu Online Library, 2008, **p. 207**).

"Blow that Breaches the Sky, The," (通天搥, Mandarin: *TONG TIAN CHUI*, Cantonese: *TUNG TIN CEOI*) – punch from down to up (similar to an uppercut in boxing) **[pp. 114, 116, 146]**.

"Bull Strikes with Its Horn, The," (牛角搥, Mandarin: *NIU JIAO CHUI*, Cantonese: *NGAU GOK CEOI*) – a circular punch delivered with the elbow bent (similar to a hook in boxing) (**Fig. 45**), **[pp. 114, 116, 146, 147]**.

C

"Covering Wing" (匝膀, Mandarin: *KAN BANG* , Cantonese: *KAM BONG*) - blocking a strike with the hand (palm), usually from top to bottom, with a "pressing" or "slapping" motion (**Fig. 81**), **[p. 188]**.

"Crane Beak, A," (鶴頂, Mandarin: *HE DING*, Cantonese: *HOK DENG*).

"Crane Wing, A," (鶴翅, Mandarin: *HE CHI*, Cantonese: *HOK CHI*).

"Crossing Palm" (橫掌, Mandarin: *HENG ZHANG*, Cantonese: *WAANG JEUNG*) - a horizontal open palm block that deflects the strike to the side **[p. 92]**.

"Crosswind Shakes the Willow" (斜風擺柳, Mandarin: *XIE FENG BAI LIU*, Cantonese: *CE FUNG BAAI LAU*) - A sweep of the enemy's leg (or both legs) with a wide circular motion of the foot. Both arms move in the opposite direction, towards the sweeping leg, enhancing the sweeping effect (**Fig. 54**), **[pp. 134, 135, 136]**.

"Cutting Bridge, A," (割橋, Mandarin: *GE QIAO*, Cantonese: *GOT KIU*) - a block (or blow) using the forearm; one of the fighting applications of the *"Stable Golden Bridge"* (定金橋) technique **[pp. 128, 129]**.

"Cutting Hand" (割手, Mandarin: *GE SHOU*, Cantonese: *GOT SAU*) - Cutting block with the edge of the palm, the movement is directed from top to bottom **[pp. 74, 86, 88, 92]**.

"Cutting with Wings" (切膀, Mandarin: *QIE BANG*, Cantonese: *CHIT BONG*) — blocking with the outer sides of the forearms from top to bottom **(Figs. 11, 47) [pp. 48, 118]**.

D

"Diagonal Downward Elbow" (睜撇, Mandarin: *ZHENG PIE*, Cantonese: *ZAANG PIT*) - the striking elbow moves in a downward diagonal path to target areas like the opponent's forehead, eyebrow, or cheek. To perform the blow, you need to raise your elbow up and to the side, approximately at the level of the forehead, the hand is near the chin, and then slash it down at an angle, often incorporating body weight and rotation for power; the blow can be used to break an opponent's guard, **[pp. 150, 151]**.

"Dividing the Gold Bridge" (分金橋, Mandarin: **FEN JIN QIAO**, Cantonese: **FAN GAM KIU**) - a movement as if tearing some cloth, the effort is burst-like, the blow is delivered with the back of your fist or with your forearm **[pp. 8, 58, 77, 128]**.

"Do a Mark with a Piercing Hand" (標串掌, Mandarin: **BIAO CHUAN ZHANG**, Cantonese: **BIU CYUN JEUNG**) - a thrust blow with the ends of fingers of an open palm **[pp. 36, 56, 66, 70, 84, 86, 88, 90, 126, 180]**.

"Double Attack with Arms Like Scissors" (較剪雙攻手法, Mandarin: **JIAO JIAN SHUANG GONG SHOU FA**, Cantonese: **GAAU JIN SEUNG GUNG SAU FAAT**) - simultaneous blows with two arms in the horizontal plane **[pp. 112, 113]**.

"Double Tiger Claw" (雙虎爪, Mandarin: **SHUANG HU ZHAO**, Cantonese: **SEUNG FU ZAAU**) **[p. 144]**.

"Draw the Bow and Shoot the Arrow" (猛弓射箭, Mandarin: **MENG GONG SHE JIAN**, Cantonese: **MANG GUNG SE JIN**) - see text and commentaries to **Fig. 83**, **[pp. 134, 146, 192, 223]**.

E

"Elbow Like a Stone Pestle" (頂碌, Mandarin: **DING LU**, Cantonese: **DENG LUK**) - a straight strike with the tip of the elbow to the side, horizontally, at shoulder level **(Fig. 23)**, **[p. 150]**.

"Enter the Small Gate" means to attack the enemy at a lower level. The theory of the **Hung Gar** style identifies five directions of attack, or five **"Gates"** (門, Cantonese: **MUN**), through which one can enter the enemy's defense space. Those are the upper, lower, and middle levels, as well as the left and right sides **[p. 126]**.

"Entwining Skill" (纏技, Mandarin: **CHAN JI**, Cantonese: **CIN GEI**) - deflecting block against a kick **(Fig. 53)**, **[p. 133, 134, 135]**.

F

"Fierce Tiger Lurking Under a Rock, The," (猛虎隱巖, Mandarin: **MENG HU YING YANG**, Cantonese: **MAANG FU JAN NGAAM**) — dodging an enemy attack by moving to a low **SEI PING MAA** stance with a deflecting block with the elbow and forearm **(Figs. 44, 59)**, **[pp. 114, 144]**.

Five Elements (五行, Mandarin: ***WU XING***, Cantonese: ***NG HANG***) - the five primordial (basic) elements, a fundamental concept in Chinese philosophy and cosmology: **Wood**, **Fire**, **Earth**, **Metal**, and **Water [p. 76]**.

"Flying Crane, A," (飛鶴, Mandarin: ***FEI HE***, Cantonese: ***FEI HOK***).

"Four Fingers Support the Sky" (四指撐天, Mandarin: ***SI ZHI CHENG TIAN***, Cantonese: ***SEI ZI CAANG TIN***) - four of your fingers are completely straight and spread wide with effort, the thumb is perpendicular to the palm plane and directed forward. Your wrists are bent toward the outer side of your forearms. You should feel some tension in your wrists, thumbs, and fingers. This is one of the basic exercises for strengthening hands, fingers and forearms **[pp. 38, 128]**.

G

"Gold-Splitting Fist, The," (分金拳, Mandarin: ***FEN JIN QUAN***, Cantonese: ***FAN GAM KYUN***) - Pull your fist toward the center of your chest, then lower your fist out to the side to waist level. In the final position, the back of the fist faces the earth, the elbow is slightly bent and placed near the side, and the forearm is in a horizontal plane. **[pp. 76, 77, 94]**.

"Golden Dragon Presents Its Claws" (金龍爪獻, Mandarin: *JIN LONG ZHAO XIAN*, Cantonese: *GAM LUNG ZAAU HIN*) - turn toward the attacking opponent with a sweeping block with both forearms in a horizontal plane; hands in a "claw" position; the twisting force of the lower back is used, which enhances the blocking motion of the forearms **(Fig. 85)**, **[p. 196]**.

H

"Hand Breaking a Line, The," (破排手, Mandarin: ***PO PAI SHOU***, Cantonese: ***PO PAI SAU***) - Circle and push blocking movements with palms and forearms, which can be performed in a vertical, horizontal, or diagonal direction **[pp. 50, 51, 56, 108, 112]**.

"Hand Coiling Around a Branch" (纏枝手, Mandarin: ***CHAN ZHI SHOU***, Cantonese: ***CIN ZI SAU***) - a deflecting block with a possible subsequent grab of the opponent's arm; performed by "coiling" hand movement around the forearm of the opponent's attacking arm **[pp. 198, 200, 202]**.

"Hand Like a Wing, A," (翅手, Mandarin: *CHI SHOU*, Cantonese: *CHI SAU*) - an outside block with the edge of the palm to deflect a strike away from the defender and across the attacker **[pp. 40, 42]**.

"Hand of 1000 Characters, The," (千字手, Mandarin: *QIAN ZI SHOU*, Cantonese: *CIN JI SAU*) - a wide range of blows and blocking with the arm (forearm), both from the inside out and the outside in, at different angles to the line of attack. The variations of this technique are shown in **Figs. 29, 35, 38, 42 [pp. 48, 66, 82, 84, 106, 110, 138, 140, 150, 151, 170]**. See also: Lam Sai Wing, *Tiger and Crane,* **Fig. 49.**

"Hand of the Golden Dragon" (金龍手, Mandarin: *JIN LONG SHOU*, Cantonese: *GAM LUNG SAU*) – a complex deflecting block technique that allows you to parry almost any enemy attack on all three levels (upper, middle and lower) **[p. 174]**.

"Hand Restraining the Tiger" (伏虎手) *FU HU SHOU (Mandarin)*, *FOOK FU SAU (Cantonese)* - a technique for gripping an attacking arm of the enemy by the wrist region followed by pressure, from up to down, with the palm to an elbow joint in the direction opposite to its natural curve. This technique and its combat application are described in detail by **Lam Sai Wing** in *Tiger and Crane*, where this method is called *"The Hand of Jin Gang Taming the Tiger"*. *Jin Gang (Mandarin)*, 金刚, (*Cantonese:* *Gaam Gong, Sanskrit: Vajrapani*) - a guard of Buddhist temples, an "Iron Warrior" **[pp. 30, 32]**.

"Hanging Foot Stance" (馬吊腳, Mandarin: *MA DIAO JIAO*, Cantonese: *MAA DIU GEUK*) - known in modern *WUSHU* as the *"Cat's Stance"* (**Fig. 26**). The term *"MAA"* is used in the meaning "a stance" here **[pp. 80, 82, 98, 100, 102, 112, 130, 132, 140, 189, 200, 201, 202, 208, 210]**.

"Hide the Flower in the Sleeve" (袖裏藏花, Mandarin: *XIU GUO ZONG HUA*, Cantonese: *ZAU GWO CONG FAA*) - a blow with the heel of an open hand, fingers turned outward, **Fig. 80, [pp. 184, 185, 186, 198]**.

"Hook Spring Leg" (拘彈脚, Mandarin: *ZU TAN JIAO*, Cantonese: *KEOI TAAN GEUK*), the same as the *"Three-Star Hook Spring Leg"* (三星鉤彈腳, Mandarin: *SAN SING ZHU TAN JIAO*, Cantonese: *SAAM SING*

KAU TAAN GEUK) - a low sweeping kick with the shin (lower shinbone), hooking and sweeping of the front-standing leg of the enemy, followed by a kick to the knee or ankle of his supporting leg or a reverse leg sweep **[pp. 192, 194, 226]**.

Horse Riding Stance (四平馬, Mandarin: ***SEI PING MA***, Cantonese: ***SEI PING MAA***) – literally: ***"Four Levels Horse Stance"***, also known as the ***"Horse Stance"*** (馬步, *MA BU*) **[pp. 46, 58, 62, 70, 80, 114, 134, 146, 174, 186, 192]**.

"Hungry Crane, A," (餓鶴, Mandarin: *E HE*, Cantonese: *NGO HOK*).

"Hungry Tiger Catches the Sheep, The," (餓虎擒羊, Mandarin: ***E HU QIN YANG***, Cantonese: ***NGO FU KAM YEUNG***) means to grip an enemy's arm in the wrist region with one hand and sharply pull to yourself and down. Simultaneously, with the forearm of another arm, using body weight, press on the elbow of the gripped hand in the direction opposite its natural curve **[p. 40]**. This technique is described in detail by **Lam Sai Wing** in *Tiger and Crane*, **Fig. 61**.

I

"Iron Hand of the Buddhist Tutor, The," (鉄臂禪師, Mandarin: ***ZHI BI CHAN SHI***, Cantonese: ***TIT BEI SIM SI***) - a set of special exercises for developing the strength of the hands and fingers, practiced in the **Southern Shaolin** styles. Mastering these methods enables one to deliver powerful blows with a "tiger paw" and execute effective grabs **(p. 38)**.

J

JI NG BAAT FAN MAA (子午八分馬, Mandarin: ***ZI WU BA FEN MA***, Cantonese: ***JI NG BAAT FAN MAA***) – literally: ***"Four Levels JI NG Stance"*** - lower ***"Bow and Arrow"*** stance, i.e., the feet are widespread, the center of gravity is situated low (**Fig. 36**), **[p. 96]**.

JI NG MAA (子午馬, Mandarin: ***ZI WU MA***, Cantonese: ***JI NG MAA***) - known in the modern *WUSHU* as the stance ***"Bow and Arrow"*** (**Fig. 19**). The term ***"MAA"*** is used in the meaning "a stance" here.

K

"Kitten Washes Its Muzzle, The," (貓兒洗面, Mandarin: *MAO ER XI MIAN*, Cantonese: *MAAU JI SAI MIN*) – Scratching motion with both hands from top to bottom and towards you. One arm is slightly extended forward, and the second hand is located at the elbow of the first. Attacking the opponent's face with the "tiger's claws" while simultaneously blocking his counter-punch (**Fig. 36**) **[pp. 96, 98, 100, 102]**.

L

"Leopard Fist" (豹拳, Mandarin: *BAO QUAN*, Cantonese: *PAAU KYUN*) - the four fingers are bent at the first phalangeal joint to expose the fore-knuckles as the striking surface, rather than the knuckles; the thumb is tucked closely against the side of the hand **[p. 138]**.

"Lock the Iron Gate with a Bolt Weighing 1000 Jin" (鐵門閂槌千斤, Mandarin: *TIE MEN SHUAN CHUI QIAN JIN*, Cantonese: - *TIT MUN SAAN CHEUI CIN GAN*) - a technique that has various applications, which are described later in this book (see **Fig. 82**), as well as in **Lam Sai Wing**'s book *Tiger and Crane*, **Fig. 59**. In this case, it refers to a simultaneous punch with both fists, from the bottom up, with an upward movement, aimed at the opponent's stomach and neck (or chin). *Jin* (Cantonese: *Gan*, 斤) is a traditional Chinese unit for weight. One *Jin* is approximately equal to 1.316 lb (600 grams) **[pp. 42, 43, 138, 188, 190]**.

"Look at Yourself in a Hand Mirror" (照鏡手法, Mandarin: *ZHAO JING SHOU FA*, Cantonese: *ZIU GENG SAU FAAT*) – a blocking movement with the side of the forearm from the inside to outside, in the final phase the palm is open and placed in front of your face (**Fig. 35**), **[pp. 96, 98, 102]**.

O

"Overhanging Blow and Punch" (掛打搥, Mandarin: *GUA DA CHUI*, Cantonese: *GWA DAA CEOI*) - the technique involves two blows performed one after the other: the *GWA* (掛拳, *"Overhanging Fist"*, **see index p. 222**) with the front hand, followed by a *CEOI* (搥, straight punch) with the back hand.

"Overhanging Fist" (掛拳, Mandarin: **GUA QUAN**, Cantonese: **GWA KYUN**) - blow (or a block) with the back side of the fist and (or) the outer side of the forearm delivered from up to down. The fist moves from the shoulder level to the waist, making a semi-circle in the vertical plane **[pp. 94, 104, 164, 166, 172, 182, 206, 215, 222]**.

P

"Pair of Cutting Wings, A," (雙切膀, Mandarin: **SHUANG QIE BANG**, Cantonese: **SEUNG CHIT BONG**) - simultaneous blocking with both arms of an enemy's attack at the upper and the middle level with using *"Arm Like a Wing"* (膀手, **BANG SHOU**), **Figs.41, 56, [108, 138]**.

"Pair of Hands like Wings, A," (雙翅手, Mandarin: **SHUANG CHI SHOU**, Cantonese: **SEUNG CHI SAU**) - an outside block with the edges of palms to deflect a strike away from the defender and across the attacker **[p. 32]**.

"Pair of Wings Cut as Knives" (雙膀插, Mandarin: **SHUANG BANG CHA**, Cantonese: **SEUNG BONG CAAP**) - a block with two arms, from top to bottom, against a blow to the lower part of the body **(Fig. 55 - rear view, Fig. 40 - front view), [p. 136]**.

"Paired Overhanging Blows from Up to Down" (掛搥雙落, Mandarin: **GUA CHUI SHUANG LUO**, Cantonese: **GWA CEOI SEUNG LOK**) - simultaneous blows (or a block) with the backsides of both fists and (or) the outer sides of forearms delivered from up to down. The fists move from the forehead level forward and down to the chest level **[p. 112]**. The same as the *"Paired Overhanging Fist"* (雙掛拳).

"Paired Overhanging Fist" (雙掛拳, Mandarin: **SHUANG GUA QUAN**, Cantonese: **SEUNG GWA KYUN**) - simultaneous blows (or a block) with the backsides of both fists and (or) the outer sides of forearms delivered from up to down. The fists move from the forehead level forward and down to the chest level **[pp. 66, 106, 110, 112, 142]**.

"Paired Work of 1000 Characters" (雙工千字, Mandarin: **SHUANG GONG QIAN ZI**, Cantonese: **SEUNG GUNG CHIN JI**) - Simultaneous action with both arms: one arm blocks the opponent's strike at the top level with a bottom-up movement, the other hand blocks (or strikes) at the middle level with a horizontal movement **[pp. 48, 140]**.

"Palms like Butterflies" (蝶掌, Mandarin: *DIE ZHANG*, Cantonese: *DIP JEUNG*) - circular block with both palms in the frontal plane, followed by a simultaneous blow with open palms at two levels, the fingers of the upper palm are directed upwards, the fingers of the lower palm are directed downwards **(Figs. 52, 63, 66, 89)**, **[pp. 44, 50, 130, 132, 152, 156, 158, 204, 206]**.

"Phoenix Eye Fist" (鳳眼拳, Mandarin: *FENG YAN QUAN*, Cantonese: *FUNG NGAAN KYUN*) – a technique focuses the power into a single point, specifically the second joint of the curled index finger, for striking vulnerable areas like the eye, temple, throat, solar plexus, etc. **[p. 176]**.

"Piercing Bridge, The," (穿橋, Mandarin: *CHUN QIAO*, Cantonese: *CHYUN KIU*) – One of the 12 basic techniques (十二支橋, *"12 Bridges"*, *SAHP YIH JI KIU*) of the *Hung Gar* style. The hand is in the position shown in **Fig. 13**. The arm is slightly bent at the elbow and stretched forward, and the elbow is turned down and slightly lowered **[p. 46]**. See also Lam Sai Wing, *Iron Thread. Southern Shaolin Hung Gar Kung Fu Classics Series* (2008).

"Pressing Fist" (責拳, Mandarin: *ZE QUAN*, Cantonese: *ZAAK KYUN*), also known as the *"Hammer Fist"* - blow (or a block) with the forearm and (or) the bottom of the fist, the part near the little finger; delivered from top to bottom **[p. 206]**.

"Pull out Fists" (抽拳, Mandarin: *CHOU QUAN*, Cantonese: *CAU KYUN*) **[p. 34]**.

"Pulling Arrow Fist" (搯箭拳, Mandarin: *MENG JIAN QUAN*, Cantonese: *MANG JIN KYUN*), full name: *"Draw the Bow and Shoot the Arrow"* (搯弓射箭, Mandarin: *MENG GONG SHE JIAN*, Cantonese: *MANG GUNG SE JIN*) - see text and commentaries to **Fig. 83**, **[pp. 134, 146]**.

"Pushing Elbow" (迫脛, Mandarin: *PO ZHENG*, Cantonese: *BIK ZAANG*) - using the elbow to block mid- and upper-level strikes; the elbow can be pushed forward to defend against a straight blow (and damage to the opponent's striking limb), or the elbow can be used in a vertical or diagonal motion to block strikes coming from different angles **(Fig. 87)** **[pp. 198, 200, 202]**.

R

"Rising Bridge, A," (提橋, Mandarin: *TI QIAO*, Cantonese: *TAI KIU*) - a blow with the outside or side of the forearm (or fist), directed from the bottom up [p. 128].

S

"Scissor Stance" (剪馬, Mandarin: *JIAN MA*, Cantonese: *ZIN MAA*) - this position is shown in **Fig. 21**.

"Side Palm" (側掌, Mandarin: *QE ZHANG*, Cantonese: *JAK JEUNG*) - a blow with the heel of an open palm, fingers turned outward, **Fig. 31**, [**pp. 88, 184, 186**].

"Single Arm Like a Wing" (單膀手, Mandarin: *DAN BANG SHOU*, Cantonese: *DAAN BONG SAU*) - a forearm block [**pp. 62, 188, 190**].

"Single Leg Flying Crane" (獨脚飛鶴, Mandarin: *DU JIAO FEI HE*, Cantonese: *DUK GEUK FEI HOK*).

"Single Tiger Claw" (單虎爪, Mandarin: *DAN HU ZHAO*, Cantonese: *DAAN FU ZAAU*), [**p. 144**].

"Slap With the Palm to Drive a Nail" (山釘拳, Mandarin: *KAN DING QUAN*, Cantonese: *KAM DENG KYUN*) - a blow (or block) with the heel of a clenched fist; delivered from top to bottom, or from top to bottom diagonally, or in horizontal plane [**p. 255**]. There is an exercise in the hard branch of *Shaolin Qi Gong* for nailing with a hand, which probably gave the name to this technique: a big nail, abutting the center of a palm with its head and being held with the extreme phalanges of the middle and fourth finger, is driven into a board with one strike [**p. 206**].

"Snake-Shaped Hand Technique" (蛇形手法, Mandarin: *SHE XING SHOU FA*, Cantonese: *SE JING SAU FAAT*) – various fingertip strikes to vulnerable points on the enemy's body: the eyes, temples, throat, solar plexus, etc., [**pp. 178, 180**].

"Soul-Returning Hand" (還魂手, Mandarin: *HUAN HUN SHOU*, Cantonese: *WAAN WAN SAU*) - a straight punch with the rear fist in the *JI NG MAA* (*"Bow and Arrow"*) position, **Fig. 88**, [**p. 200**].

"Squeeze a Wooden Billet and Punch" (夾木拳, Mandarin: *JIA MU QUAN*, Cantonese: *GAAP MUK KYUN*) - a block with the front arm, and simultaneously punch with the rear arm. At the final stage of the strike, your elbows should be fairly close together, as if you're squeezing a wooden billet between your elbows, preventing it from falling **[pp. 162, 164]**.

"Stable Gold Bridge" (定金橋, Mandarin: ***DING JIN QIAO***, Cantonese: ***DING GAM KIU***) - the arms are extended forward at chest level, parallel to each other, but not fully straightened; elbows pointing down; four of your fingers are completely straight and spread wide with effort, the thumb is perpendicular to the palm plane and directed forward. Your wrists are bent toward the outer side of your forearms. You should feel some tension in your wrists and thumbs. This is one of the basic exercises for strengthening the forearms **[Figs. 12, 48, pp. 50, 108, 122]**. See also Lam Sai Wing, *Iron Thread. Southern Shaolin Hung Gar Kung Fu Classics Series* (2008).

"Stable Horse Riding Stance" (四平八分馬, Mandarin: ***SEI PING BA FEN MA***, Cantonese: ***SEI PING BAAT FAN MAA***) – literally: *"Four Levels Eight Parts Horse Stance"* - lower *"Horse Stance"*, i.e., the feet are widespread, the center of gravity is situated low **[pp. 62, 146, 186, 192]**.

T

"Three Openings" (三株, Mandarin: ***SAN ZHU***, Cantonese: ***SAAM ZYU***) is one of the most important basic techniques of ***Hung Gar*** style inherited from the *Southern Shaolin*. The *Shaolin "Treatises on Fighting Arts"* say: *"It is necessary to pay special attention to the fact that the Mind would guide the Breath-Qi and the Breath-Qi should act in unity with the physical Force-Li. The Breath-Qi must strengthen the physical Force-Li and the Force-Li must guide the Breath-Qi"*. This, in outward appearance, a simple exercise, is aimed at training the said cooperation. The hands are in a position of *"One Finger"* (*JAT ZI*), as shown in **Fig. 13**. The initial position: the palms are on the shoulder level, and the elbows are lowered on the sides. Take a sharp breath in through the mouth and "close" *Qi* (strain your stomach and hold breathing), then slowly, with an effort, pull the palms aside on the shoulder level. **[pp. 36, 38, 52, 54, 124]**.

"Three-Star Hook Spring Leg" (三星鉤彈腳, Mandarin: **SAN XING ZHU TAN JIAO**, Cantonese: **SAAM SING KAU TAAN GEUK**) - a low sweeping kick with the shin (lower shinbone), hooking and sweeping of the front-standing leg of the enemy, followed by a kick to the knee or ankle of his supporting leg or a reverse leg sweep **[pp. 50, 51, 126, 134, 192, 220]**.

"Throwing Fist" (拋拳, Mandarin: **PAO QUAN,** Cantonese: **PAAU KYUN**) – a blow with the back of a fist, from down to up. The arm is almost completely straightened at the elbow joint. The movement starts from the hip and is reinforced due to a turn of the body. Another arm naturally draws down and backwards. This technique can serve as a block: in this case, the outer surface of a forearm is used. The final phase of the blow is shown in **Fig. 78, [pp. 182, 215]**.

"Throwing the Elbow Up" (拋踭上, Mandarin: **PAO ZHENG SHANG**, Cantonese: **PAAU ZAANG SOENG**) – blocking (or blow) with the elbow from bottom to top, in the final phase, the arm is completely bent, the hand is located near the temple, the elbow is at the level of the chin **(Fig. 46), [pp. 116, 118]**.

"Tiger Descends from the Mountain" (下山虎, Mandarin: **XIA SHAN HU**, Cantonese: **HAA SAAN FU**) - This technique is described in detail by **Lam Sai Wing** in *Tiger and Crane*, **Fig. 63, [p. 144]**.

"Tiger Hiding in the Mountains" (隱山虎, Mandarin: **YIN SHAN HU**, Cantonese: **JAN SAAN FU**) **[p. 144]**.

"Tiger Tail Kick, The," (虎尾脚, Mandarin: **HU WEI JIAO**, Cantonese: **FU MEI GEUK**) – a side kick, powerful, linear strike delivered with the heel or the entire outside edge of the foot; usually used to hit targets like the opponent's shins, knees, groin, or rib cage **(Fig. 75), [pp. 176, 177]**.

"To Take the Horse by the Bridle and Bring It Back to the Stall" (帶馬歸槽拉, Mandarin: **DAI MA GUI CAO LA**, Cantonese: **DAAI MAA GWAI COU LAAI**) – i.e., to catch the enemy's clothes and to pull him towards yourself, at the same time to move the body back and to shift the center of gravity to the back supporting leg **[pp. 98, 100, 102, 104]**.

"Turn and Divide, Penetrate with Hands" (轉分漏手, Mandarin: *ZHUAN FEN LOU SHOU*, Cantonese: *JYUN FAN LAU SAU*) - see commentaries on **page 44**, **[pp. 44, 132, 204]**.

"Two Dragons Snatching Pearls" (二龍搶珠, Mandarin: *ER LONG QIANG ZHU*, Cantonese: *JI LUNG COENG ZYU*) — a thrust into the enemy's eyes with the tips of the index and middle fingers, the remaining fingers pressed to the center of the palm (the character 珠, in addition to representing a pearl, also signifies the pupil of the eye), **(Fig. 76)**, **[p. 178]**.

U

"Unicorn Step" (麒麟步, Mandarin: *QI LIN BU*, Cantonese: *KEI LEON BOU*) - a specific footwork technique that allows you to turn in any direction at the desired angle in two movements (steps). First, step with the back foot, placing it in front of the front foot, close to it, with knees close together, and shift the body weight forward. Then, pivot on the front foot to the desired angle and step forward with the back foot. In this form, this step is used when performing the *"Butterfly Palms"* technique to perform a 180-degree turn (two steps, one after the other). **Figs. 95, 96**, **[pp. 156, 158, 180, 182, 215]**.

"Uninterrupted Punches Like Rockets" or *"Fists like Rockets Strike one after another"* (火箭連環拳, Mandarin: *HUO JIAN LIAN HUAN QUAN*, Cantonese: *FO JIN LIN WAAN KYUN*) - a rapid succession of punches, following each other without a break, like rain drumming on a roof **[pp. 46, 192]**.

W

"Well-Fed Crane, A," (飽鶴, Mandarin: *BAO HE*, Cantonese: *BAAU HOK*).

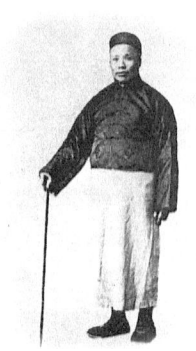

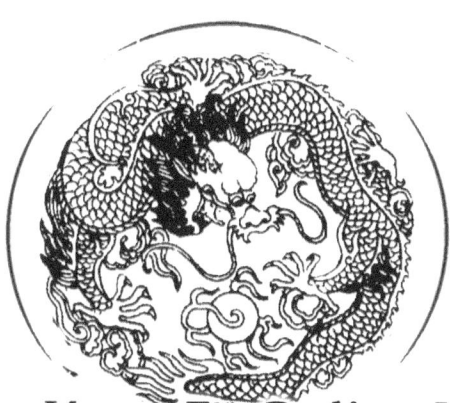

Shaolin Kung Fu Online Library
www.kungfulibrary.com

Chinese Martial Arts - Theory & Practice
Old Chinese Books, Treatises, Manuscripts

Lam Sai Wing. TAMING THE TIGER. SOUTHERN SHAOLIN HUNG GAR KUNG FU CLASSICS SERIES.

Lam Sai Wing. Tiger and Crane Double Form.

Lam Sai Wing. Iron Thread. Southern Shaolin Hung Gar Kung Fu Classics Series.

Jin Jing Zhong. Training Methods of 72 Arts of Shaolin.

Jin Jing Zhong. Dian Xue Shu: Skill of Acting on Acupoints.

Liu Jin Sheng. CHIN NA FA: Skill of Catch and Hold.

Tang Ji Ren. Pugilistic Art of the Tang Family. DA HONG QUAN.

Xu Yi Qian. CHUAN NA QUAN: Style of Piercing Blows and Holds.

Yuan Chu Cai. MEI HUA ZHUANG: Poles of Plum Blossom. External and Internal Training.

shaolinkungfulibrary.com

Southern Shaolin Hung Gar Kung Fu and Qigong
Canonical Books by Lam Sai Wing

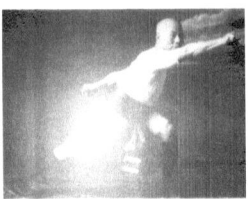

Lam Sai Wing
(1860-1943)

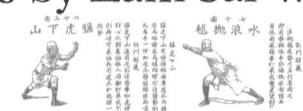

"SINCE MY YOUNG YEARS TILL NOW, FOR 50 YEARS, I HAVE BEEN LEARNING FROM MASTERS. I AM HAPPY THAT I HAVE EARNED THE LOVE OF MY TUTORS WHO PASSED ON ME THE SHAOLIN MASTERY..."

Lam Sai Wing was one of the best fighters of his time, an outstanding master of Southern Shaolin Hung Gar Kung Fu and a disciple of the legendary Wong Fei Hung. At the beginning of twentieth century, supposedly in 1917-1923, when Lam Sai Wing was the Chief Instructor in hand-to-hand combat in the armed forces of Fujian province, he wrote three books on traditional Shaolin methods of the achievement of the highest mastership. In those books he scrutinized COMBAT TECHNIQUES of TIGER and CRANE style, as well as the OLD SHAOLIN METHOD of developing the "INTERNAL" and "EXTERNAL" power. The books are illustrated with a great number of fine drawings showing the author demonstrate his wonderful techniques. Until now the books of Master Lam Sai Wing serve as a basic textbook for those who seriously practices Hung Gar in China.

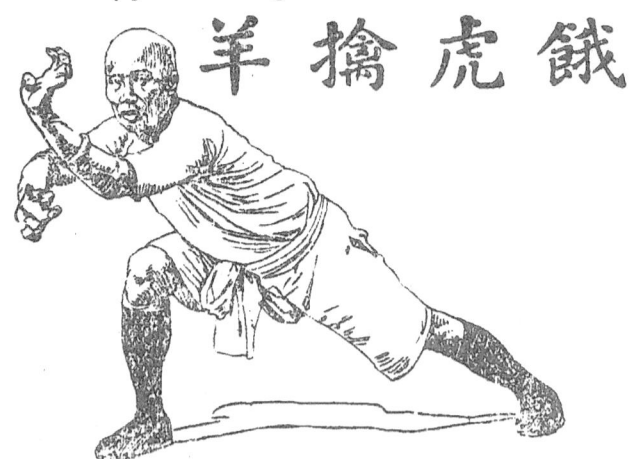

www.kungfulibrary.com

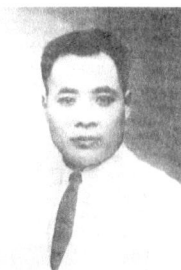 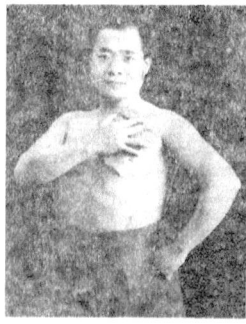 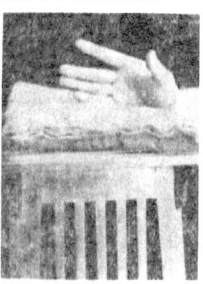
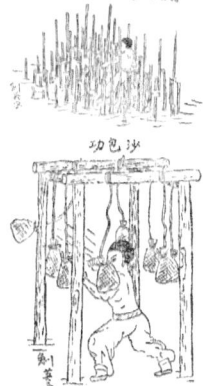

Also by Lam Sai Wing:

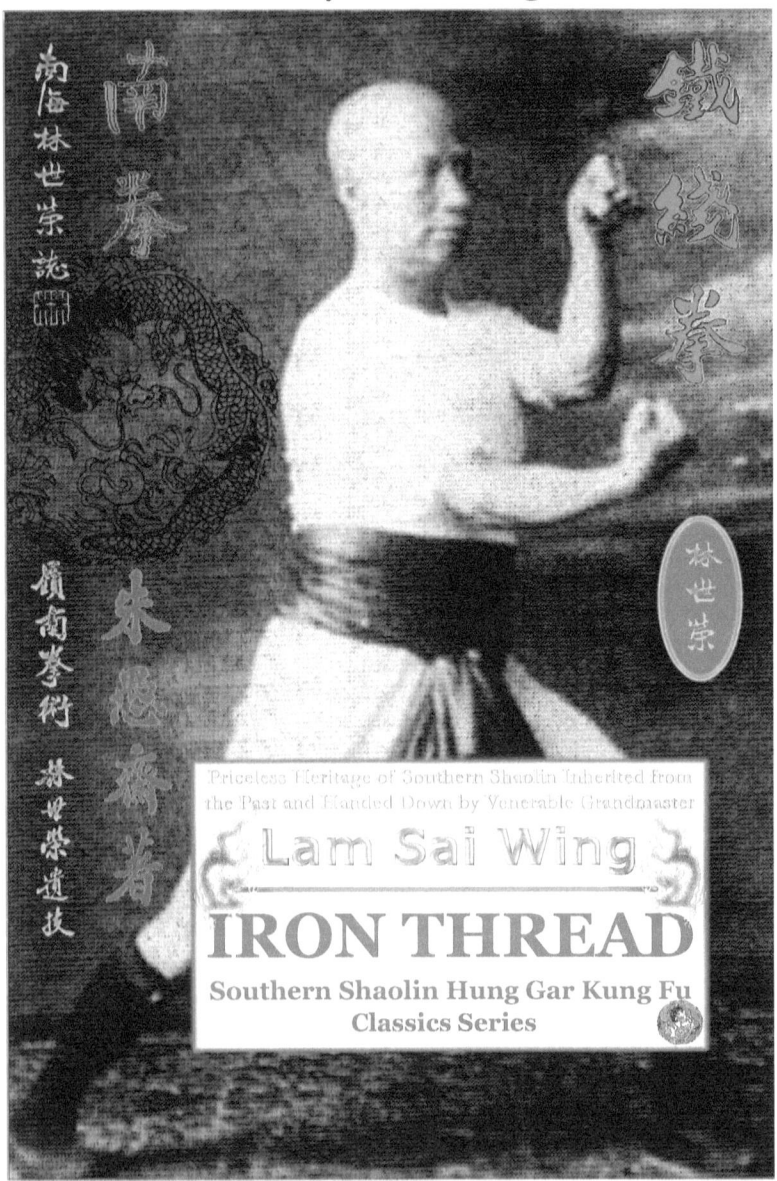

Priceless Heritage of Southern Shaolin Inherited from
the Past and Handed Down by Venerable Grandmaster

Lam Sai Wing

IRON THREAD
Southern Shaolin Hung Gar Kung Fu
Classics Series

Published by Shaolin Kung Fu Online Library

Also by Lam Sai Wing:

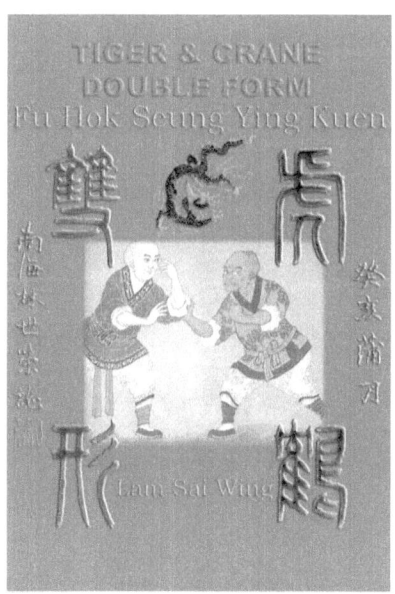

Published by Shaolin Kung Fu Online Library

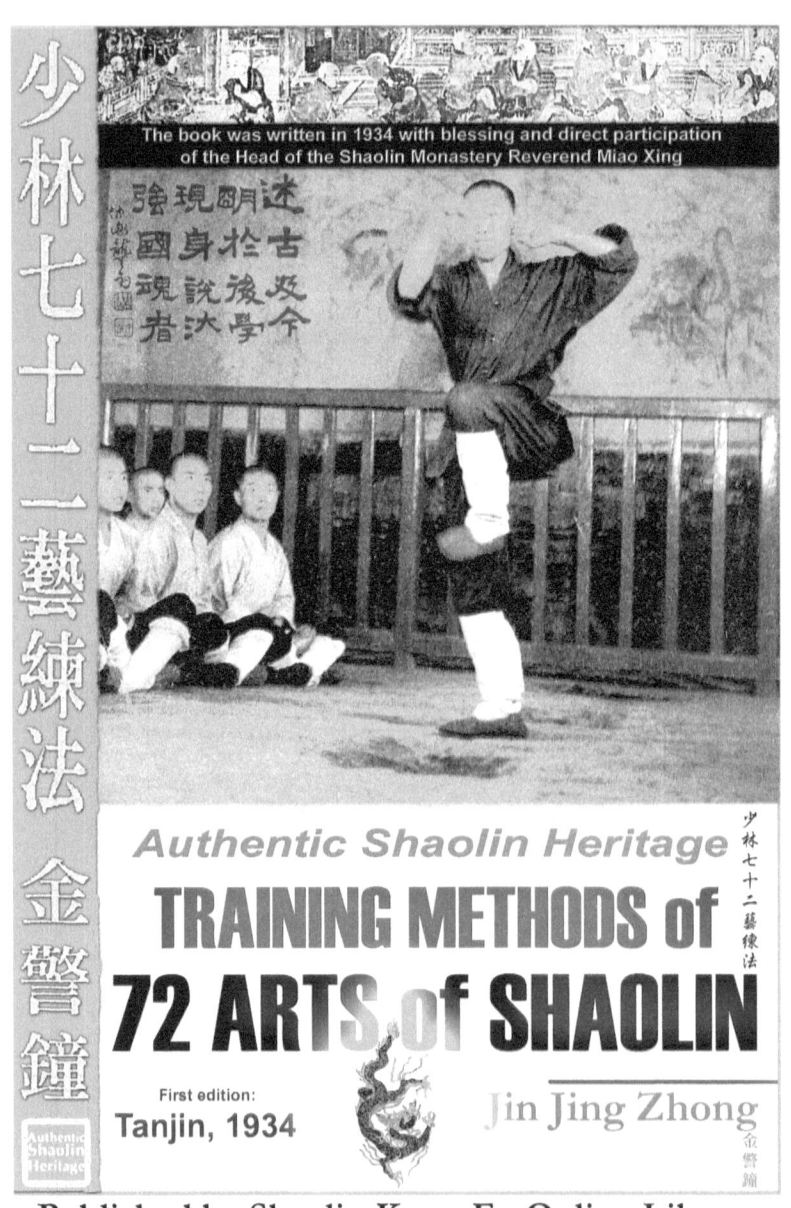

The book was written in 1934 with blessing and direct participation of the Head of the Shaolin Monastery Reverend Miao Xing

Authentic Shaolin Heritage

TRAINING METHODS of
72 ARTS of SHAOLIN

First edition:
Tanjin, 1934

Jin Jing Zhong

少林七十二藝練法金警鐘

Published by Shaolin Kung Fu Online Library

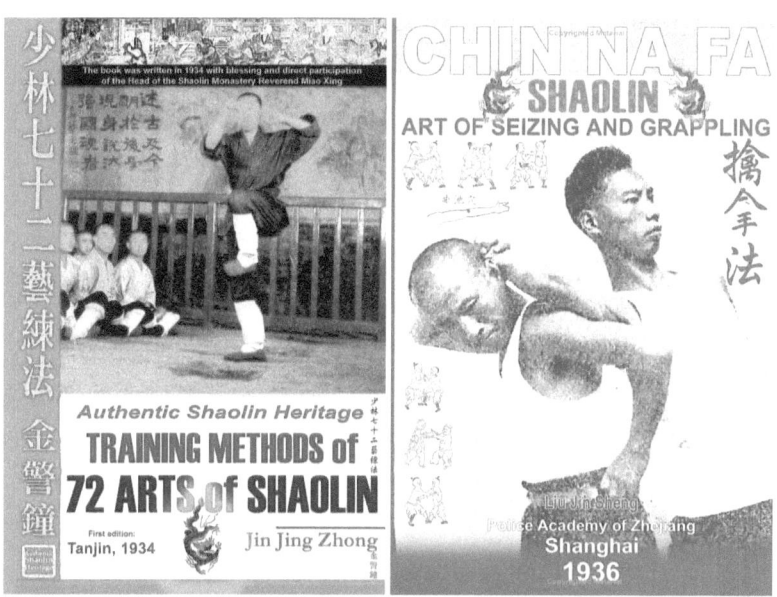

少林七十二藝練法　金警鐘

The book was written in 1934 with blessing and direct participation of the Head of the Shaolin Monastery Reverend Miao Xing

Authentic Shaolin Heritage
TRAINING METHODS of
72 ARTS of SHAOLIN
First edition:
Tanjin, 1934
Jin Jing Zhong

CHIN NA FA
SHAOLIN
ART OF SEIZING AND GRAPPLING
擒拿手法

Police Academy of Zhejiang
Shanghai
1936

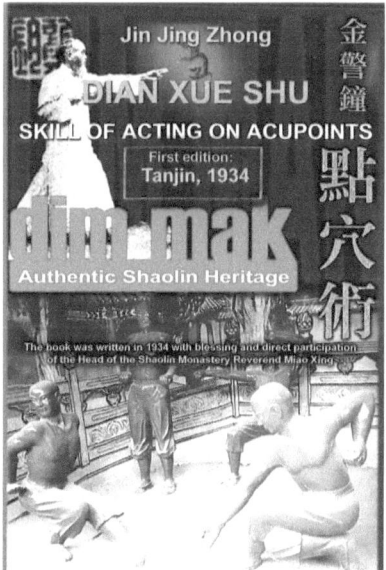

Jin Jing Zhong　金警鐘
DIAN XUE SHU
SKILL OF ACTING ON ACUPOINTS
First edition:
Tanjin, 1934
dim-mak
Authentic Shaolin Heritage
The book was written in 1934 with blessing and direct participation of the Head of the Shaolin Monastery Reverend Miao Xing
點穴術

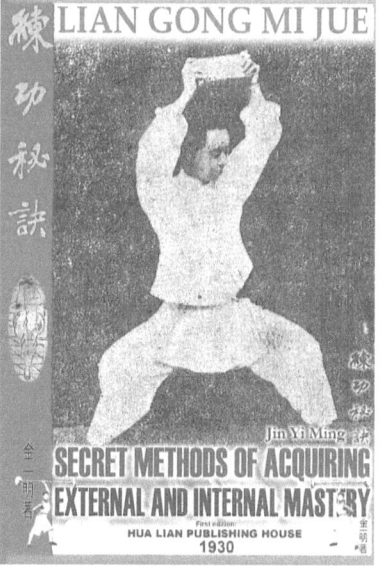

LIAN GONG MI JUE
練功秘訣

Jin Yi Ming
SECRET METHODS OF ACQUIRING
EXTERNAL AND INTERNAL MASTERY
First edition:
HUA LIAN PUBLISHING HOUSE
1930

Published by Shaolin Kung Fu Online Library

www.ingramcontent.com/pod-product-compliance
Lightning Source LLC
Chambersburg PA
CBHW020231130626
46549CB00005B/1843